Brett poignantly shares her battle with fertility, which far too often remains a silent struggle layered with social stigmas, hidden loss, and isolation. She turns her journey of pain and challenge into one of candid connection and offers invaluable hope, insight, and inspiration for anyone navigating a painful path to parenthood.

—MOIRA FORBES, EXECUTIVE VICE PRESIDENT, FORBES MEDIA; PUBLISHER, *FORBESWOMAN*

A bracingly honest story about navigating the emotional maze of infertility and IVF—this book will make you belly laugh, burst into tears, and cheer loudly all at once. Brett takes you on her journey, but what you get in return is support for your own. This is a must read for anyone experiencing infertility, and it's the book I wish I had when I went through it myself.

—JAMIE WEBBER, EDITORIAL DIRECTOR, HEALTHLINE PARENTHOOD

Brett's refreshingly witty and unapologetically honest account of her journey is absolutely worth reading. Her ability to make it fun to read is a gift. I'm so glad she was brave enough to share her story and in doing so, reduce the isolation and frustration for others who are understandably shocked when they find themselves in the same position.

—KATHLEEN HONG, MD, HCLD, ASSOCIATE DIRECTOR, RMANJ EMBRYOLOGY LABORATORY

THE UNDERWEAR IN MY SHOE

the underwear *in my* shoe

MY JOURNEY THROUGH IVF, *UNFILTERED*

BRETT RUSSO

HOUNDSTOOTH
PRESS

THE UNDERWEAR IN MY SHOE

My Journey Through IVF, Unfiltered

ISBN   978-1-5445-1463-5 *Hardcover*

978-1-5445-1462-8 *Paperback*

978-1-5445-1461-1 *Ebook*

FOR THE WOMEN GOING THROUGH IT:

YOU ARE NOT ALONE.

CONTENTS

CHAPTER 1

GOMOS

(GIRLS OBSESSED WITH MARRIAGE AND OFFSPRING)

I didn't start off obsessed with the idea of having a baby. Quite the opposite. I used to have disdain for "girls obsessed with marriage and offspring." You know the girl. The one who had a wedding Pinterest page before she even had a boyfriend. I grew up with two brothers, and for years I would watch females throwing themselves at one of them, regardless of whether my brothers showed any interest or not. Seeing these women willing to give up everything real about themselves to be the girl they thought my brothers wanted them to be always bothered me. I saw it time and time again. They would linger around for a last-minute invite to a wedding. Accepting inconsistent texts and Tuesday night plans because they didn't want to be "that girl" who asked where they stood. That girl? You mean the girl who stands up for herself?

From an early age, I knew that would never be me. As I grew up, these same girls seemed to be the ones crying to strangers in bathrooms across the West Village about not being engaged yet to their longtime boyfriends. The same girls who "lived in Manhattan" only to fake a career long enough to find a rich husband to have blonde babies with. You know them. You see them on Facebook in portraits in fields, next to barns, humblebragging their way through your news feed.

I spent a good part of my single life determined not to become "that girl." This was my city, too. The city where powerful women have careers and wear killer heels with red soles they bought themselves. Women who write important emails while walking down the sidewalk. So what if we are approaching thirty...then thirty-five...then forty. We are women of the new age. We have gay friends and get bonuses at work and won't become victim to society's views of where we should be at this stage in our lives. We are the girls who don't settle for a man we don't love just to say we have a husband, and we sure as hell don't get down when we can't get pregnant right away. We have much more going on in our lives than to be obsessed with that. Right?

I should make a confession of my own. I moved to lower Manhattan seven years ago. I have spent every day since trying to be the New Yorker I always dreamed of being. I grew up in New Jersey, and my family would always go into the city to see Broadway shows and the Rockefeller Center Christmas tree during the holidays. I would get so excited knowing we were going in. People who lived in Manhattan seemed like they were part of some cool world where people wore big sunglasses painted in brands that no one had ever heard of before. That same obsession led me to say for years that I lived in Manhattan when in actuality I lived in New Jersey. I could usually get away with it until I was caught off guard by a closet-case city girl turned suburbanite. She'd ask me what street I lived on, and as I stumbled for a response, we'd both suddenly know my jig was up.

By the time I had started dating Jack, though, I was finally living in Manhattan in an apartment overlooking Tribeca. It was small and way too expensive, but it was mine and that was all that mattered. I was officially a New Yorker. I had a job I loved. I had a collection of high heels to die for, and I walked around with this badass swagger you could see for blocks. I married Jack a year later after a long-distance love affair from across the globe. It's been a true fairy tale...until now.

My name is Brett Russo. I'm a girl with a boy's name. A girl with the same story as you.

CHAPTER 2

THE SUMMER OF SIN

Jack and I decided to wait a year after getting married to start "trying." Jack is as logical as I am, well, *not* logical. Sometimes I think if it weren't for him, I would float away. He is as sharp as they come. He's tall and very handsome. He's a reader and a thinker. Picture banker brain and hippie heart. We had only been together a short time when we got married, and I felt like we needed time together as a couple before starting a family. Because, you know, pregnancy would happen exactly when we wanted it to, of course. This was the smart choice. The logical choice. I found myself proud about that decision. It was another example that, though I was married, I was far from a GOMO.

I don't regret that decision. Although I'd be lying if I said the thought that we should've started earlier doesn't haunt me during my darker times. It was a good year, though. We traveled. We jumped on planes for last-minute weekend getaways to Aspen and Miami. We even went to San Diego for forty-eight hours just to play golf at Torrey Pines. We bounced around seeing friends.

We drank wine on Tuesdays and had dance parties in our living room. We were the envy of all our friends anchored at home with troops of toddlers at various stages of annoying. We didn't have a care in the world. Sometimes I look back and wonder if we realized how good that felt. We were like that insurance commercial: *"We are never moving to the suburbs." "We are never having kids."* I guess I never really realized how badly I wanted that life until, suddenly, I couldn't have it.

Our "trying" season started on the last night of our final trip: Hawaii. We spent ten days drinking wine, playing golf, indulging in a second honeymoon, and celebrating the end of what we called "Our Summer of Sin." That night, we sat outside on the balcony of our hotel room after a long cork-popping dinner. The moon lit up the entire Pacific. We were just tapping into our third bottle of wine. Jerry Garcia Pandora was playing on Jack's iPhone, and the world felt like it was exactly as it should be. We sat there for hours talking about how far we had come and all that this next year was certain to bring. My husband fiddled with his iPhone, and next thing I knew, "Not with Haste" by Mumford & Sons (our wedding song) was playing from the speaker. I leaned in, and we started to kiss. We made our way toward the bed. The balcony doors were open, and a cool breeze was coming in. I could hear the waves crashing against the lava. Everything felt different. We both knew what it would mean. The point that we had been building up to all our lives. Jack held me close, and I cried. It was one of the most beautiful moments of my life.

We woke up the next morning in each other's arms. The balcony door was still open, and the sun was peeking through. "Do you think it worked?" Jack asked as he smirked at me.

"I do feel a little different. Little guy is probably swimming his ass off as we speak."

The truth was, neither of us had any idea if it had worked or not, but I really believed it had. I remember that as the last moment of true naïve bliss.

From that night on, we kept trying. The first few months weren't too bad. We were lighthearted and excited. We even joked while it was happening and made up songs. It was fun. We would have sex, then the second we were done I would throw my legs up over my head and lie there naked for twenty minutes, not one second sooner. Have you ever seen your body from that angle? I don't care who you are, it's awful. And if it's not awful, you need to put down this book immediately and go eat a hamburger. It's the first time I realized I had stretch marks on my upper side thighs where my cute bubble butt used to be. Odd place for a stretch mark, I know. But the fact that my jean size in college was 30/30 at one point, I get it. I was a field hockey player. Anyway, my husband would get dressed and start walking around the apartment, and I would lie there, naked on the couch, committed to my position. *(Sorry to anyone who has spent time on our couch.)*

As the months passed, though, so did the passion. Procreation started to feel like a job. Like the elephant in the room. That little smiley face would show its taunting grin on the ovulation stick, and I would give my husband a silent hint. What started as champagne and lingerie became "Maybe put a porn on," which became "Sooo, are we going to talk about the fact that we have to have sex tonight and neither of us are in the mood?" We would both come home from work and bring up any other topic that would keep us the safest distance away from the chore of having to have sex.

Even at this point, I knew in my heart that we would be fine. I was healthy. I never did drugs. (*That's my story, and I'm sticking to it.*) My period had come every twenty-sixth day for the past twenty-five years. I had never used birth control. But most of all, we weren't crazy psycho stressed about it, so it would be fine.

My twin brother, Vince, and his wife, Grace, had gotten married a few months earlier and decided to start trying as well. Vince and I are as close as two human beings can be. He has the most genuine heart. He's funny and smart. We have done everything together for our entire lives. We went to college together. We took over our family commercial printing company together. Every memory I have involves the two of us laughing our way through it. Whether it was moving to the city or getting married, we always seemed to be doing things at the same time. We had the same friends and spent most of our time together.

When Vince and his wife started trying to have a baby, I remember thinking how crazy my sister-in-law sounded. She was almost obsessed with it. She needed to be pregnant by thirty-five for whatever reason. It was relentless. I looked down on her a little for that at the time. She was already taking prenatal vitamins and making appointments with doctors. Classic GOMO. I think at one point in some alcohol-induced moment of cattiness, I even lied and told her that prenatal vitamins would make her fat.

It would happen—for all of us. But probably us first because we weren't stressed about it. But when Vince and Grace announced that she got pregnant after their first try, I immediately started to panic. It was as if a switch was flipped inside me. Not because I wasn't happy for them. I was. But because I felt a worry that I never had before. I felt an intense need to push the fast-forward button. Wasn't I supposed to get pregnant first? We were the ones who said we would start trying first. We were the ones who got married first.

I put on an excited face and jumped up and down and hugged them. But I couldn't hide the panic. I'll never forget the look in Vince's eyes when they told me. He was almost uncomfortable. I could see that he wanted to make sure that I was okay while still trying to soak in what had just happened for him. I would be right behind him. And like everything else, we were going to start this next adventure side by side.

Then everyone around me became pregnant. I had made it through like seventeen years without seeing a pregnant woman, and now everyone I knew was farting into the wind in the right direction and getting pregnant. Hearing all the good news started to become annoying, then sickening, then embarrassing, and then completely isolating. I found myself having to field questions from unknowing bystanders. "So, when are you going to start? Time's a ticking." As if the thought that maybe I was having a problem never entered their minds. I'd answer, "Oh I don't know, soon hopefully." I mean, what did they think that I wanted to just wait it out until the last possible second before my ovaries dry up forever? You know, live on the edge.

With each passing month, I counted down the days until I could check the next pregnancy test. In the beginning, I would go into the bathroom, pee on the stick, and let it sit. While it was deciding my fate, I would grab my husband. We would slowly approach the test, careful not to sneak an accidental peek, close our eyes, count to three, and then look together. It was a cute ritual. Until, well, it wasn't anymore. Talk about an awkward silence. Seeing the disappointment in his eyes crushed me every time. As if I was failing him. I know that doesn't make any logical sense, but by then I'd thrown logic way out the window.

I started to check the test earlier and earlier each month. I would search for the test that gave me the earliest results. You know the one on the Duane Reade shelf that promised you what no other would: the sixth day. "Find out six days before your missed period." It was like the holy land. If I could just make it to that day. But like clockwork, it would come up negative and then the excuses and justifications would start. *Well, they can be wrong. It's too early to tell.* I would convince myself that it was still a possibility and search the internet until I got confirmation. I even started sneaking the tests in random public bathrooms so that my husband wouldn't know. He would beg me to wait. It was just getting too traumatic.

We bought all of the tests, one after the other. The test showing a single pink line was the least invasive. One line you aren't pregnant, two lines you are. Simple enough. But when I started seeing imaginary lines on the screen, I knew we had to switch. But the next test's "Not Pregnant" left me feeling defensive, like, "You don't know me!" Nothing was as bad though as the one that launched the abrupt word "NO" at you. It might as well have told me to go fuck myself. It always felt so insensitive.

I don't know what I expected. Maybe a little image of a fist pointing upward as if to say, "Not quite this time, but keep trying, champ." No matter which test I used, the negative result was devastating. The death of another month. The unsolidified pregnancy symptoms exposed as phantoms in my head. I had the routine down. Take the test. Get depressed. Hold on to hope. Get my period. Lose the hope. Cry. Repeat. This went on for almost a year. After the tenth month, I knew it was time to get help. It was time for Cheng.

CHAPTER 3

CHENG

You don't know 940 Tenth Avenue until you know it well. It's a huge high-rise building with big black windows going all the way up to the sky in the heart of midtown Manhattan. It had two dueling delis on either side of its entrance, both claiming to have the best pizza in New York. At 8:10 a.m., the sidewalk out front was filled with buttoned-up young professionals dressed just crisply enough to hide their hangovers from the night before. I walked into the lobby, where the bustle and confusion resembled the toy aisle in Target the week before Christmas. Some excitement, some anger, some frantic rushing, and some lingerers clinging onto their last few minutes of freedom before they headed upstairs to work.

My husband and I, who couldn't quite find the words to say to each other that morning, waited in line before the security desk. I tucked the bottom of my silk blouse into my wool skirt as I tried to blend in with the professional crowd around me. "Do you know where we're going?" Jack asked.

"Of course I know where we are going! You really think I wouldn't know?" I barked back defensively.

What was he implying? Of course I knew. I mean, this was huge. Did he really think I would be that clueless?

I snuck my hand into my pocket and tried to catch a sly glimpse of my phone to check the information. Fine, I had no idea where we were going. But he didn't need to know that.

We walked toward the desk like we were approaching the bench in a courtroom. The security guard was an older, heavyset man. He bristled with enough intimidation and pride that you knew it was not going to be an easy transaction. "What's your name?" he asked without even looking up.

I stated my name, and then he asked what company I was going to see. I briefly looked around to see if anyone was listening and then whispered, "NYCM."

He kept his eyes glued to the keyboard and merely repeated in a heavier deep voice, "Which company?" as if it were his first day on the job and he didn't recognize the name.

I moved my head slightly closer to his and whispered, "The doctor."

He looked up immediately, to catch a quick glance of the circus character I felt like: damaged goods. "Oh, one of those" is what he was probably thinking. With this doctor's office, everyone knows why you are there. You didn't just decide to stop in and get a few hundred blood tests and eighty-seven ultrasounds because hey, why not? Insurance covers merely a third of it. No, I wasn't here to start my day and set the world on fire like the other women passing by. I wasn't on my way upstairs with a little muffin in a brown paper bag to eat while checking my morning emails. Not me. Not today. Today, I was here to figure out why the hell my uterus won't do the one job it's supposed to actually do! My reaction obviously had nothing to do with my elevated level of sensitivity toward the topic.

The guard clicked on his computer a few times and then told me to smile. As I looked up, still mortified from having made this appointment, he snapped a photo of me. A picture? Really? As if this interaction couldn't be any more embarrassing. A picture that would be etched in the NYCM computer system for the rest of time as we know it. The little black-and-white label lasered with my face slid through the ID machine. I looked like a combination of petrified and roofied. Then I saw the words below the picture, "Brett Russo, Infertility Clinic." And there it would remain. In the system, forever. I quickly crushed it deep into my jacket pocket, and we headed inside.

At least the office waiting room was nice—cleaner than most NYC medical facilities I had seen. A long row of gray leather couches lined the walls all the way down to the window. The white marble coffee tables in front of each of them were filled with trashy celebrity magazines that were sure to offer the proper distractions needed while waiting. I glanced around to scope out the competition. I might as well have entered the thirty-sixth floor of the Citibank building headquarters. Women in front of their laptops, tapping away, taking calls, and doing business as usual. In a way, it made me feel empowered. These were women who worked really hard and waited to have children. I liked that for some reason. I don't think that anyone totally feels comfortable being in this sort of waiting room, but at least I felt like I was surrounded by a savvy group of women. For now, of course. I mean these women that had "issues." I wasn't one of them. I was barely supposed to be here. I was just being proactive. Spotting a little fridge with bottles of water in it, my husband grabbed his first of many "$300 bottles of water," as he would come to call them, and we waited for our name to be announced.

As the clock struck 8:30 a.m., Dr. Cheng came out of the doorway, not a second tardy. She was petite and well dressed. I noticed her trendy shoes right away, which made me intrigued with her from the start. "You must be Brett and Jack, I'm Dr. Cheng."

She was the perfect combination of warm and fierce. I took to her immediately. In a failed effort to connect, I answered, "Yes, although I bet it's hard to know if Brett's the girl or Brett's the boy."

She looked at me oddly, trying to decipher if what I said was meant to be a joke. "How about we go inside, shall we?"

Whoops. I guess I read that one wrong. "Yes, yes, of course."

We took a seat in her office, and the questions began. She started with me first. Once she started, she didn't stop. Spraying me with loaded question after loaded question as I scurried for answers, feeling like my squeaky-clean past didn't feel so squeaky-clean anymore. She asked me everything from when I got my period to my sexual history. Rabid skeletons freed from the closet en masse. I thought the first time my husband saw me on a toilet was bad. Little did I know I would be on the stand in the middle of my own personal trial.

It was an eye-opening experience. For the first time, I realized how much my age affected the process. I went from feeling like the exception to the textbook definition of the rule. I never felt so old in my entire life. Thirty-five is the age where the doctors consider you "high risk." The golden era of "advanced maternal age." "Elderly gravida." "Completely fucked."

More scientifically, it's the rookie year of the deterioration of your eggs. Every two years moving forward puts you in a deeper category of risk. Deeper into the shit storm per se. As you can imagine, walking in at thirty-eight made me feel panicked. Where the hell were the billboards telling me this when I was twenty-nine? Where was the little pamphlet from my gynecologist? "Enjoy Family Planning—unless you're over thirty-five and then you're pretty much screwed. *Free Tinder membership for your husband to meet someone younger on your way out.*"

I learned more in those thirty minutes than I had in thirty years. I was terrified. It made me want to go back in time and drop-kick my high school health teacher—to go back and listen to my mother, who told me to freeze my eggs like a bazillion years ago. Would it have killed me to ask about it? I've Googled "orangutans having sex" but never thought to Google fertility.

Cheng started to ask me a lot of questions about my mother. Evidently, heredity plays a key role in predicting the future of my own cycle. My mother is a young sixty-four. She is in perfect health. She got pregnant with my brother and me the first time she ever had sex, I think. I knew this would finally be a check in the right column for me.

"When did your mother go through menopause?" Cheng asked as she nestled back in her chair and brought her hands together. I had no idea. I had never thought to ask her. I texted her to find out. The answer to this question was vital. As we waited with bated breath for her reply, Cheng tried to lighten the mood.

"How did you guys meet?"

Jack swooped in with a heartfelt tone, "We first met in college but didn't talk again for fifteen years. We actually started writing emails to each other for months after we got reacquainted on Facebook. I was living in Hong Kong, and Brett was here in the city. The emails became like novels, and we really fell in love on paper before anything else."

Okay, that was romantic and I'm being an asshole, but really? Now he's divulging the details of our love story? He seemed so relaxed with his response. Were these two really able to swap small talk at a time like this? Was I alone in my inability to stay focused on anything other than the return text from my mother? All eyes were on that phone. It buzzed and lit up. Moment of truth. The news that would get me off the hook. And then I read it. My heart stopped. I looked up at my husband and then up at Cheng and read, "Missed one period at thirty-eight."

The silence in the room was deafening. The phone buzzed again, and in a desperate attempt to get as much info to the doctor, I started reading the text out loud before I had the chance to read it myself. "However, I was going through a rough patch emotionally with your father, and I lost forty pounds in a matter of months. Can that affect it? I didn't actually go through menopause until forty-eight. I got my period at twelve. Anyway, are you coming over for dinner later?"

The relief was so real that it should've had its own chair in the room. After a good laugh, we forged ahead.

The questions went on and on. Cheng was all business and wasted no time in between questions. I felt like I had just finished a boot camp class in the park. *(Never done that, FYI, but for a second, I bet you thought I was a real badass.)*

We moved on to Jack. Evidently, the man's equivalent to the woman's eighty-seven questions was two. Have you ever impregnated a woman before, and do you have any STDs? Seriously? I jumped to the front of my chair. "That's it? That's all you need to ask him?" You must need to know more than that. He's done things, Cheng. Oh, he's done lots of things. Tell her, Jack, tell her about all the... things. But none of that mattered—nothing except for me, my age, and my rotting eggs.

In an effort to educate us, Cheng walked us through a generic PowerPoint presentation about all of the stages of a woman's reproductive cycle and all of the risks as she gets older. It was filled with charts and statistics—all information that would've been quite useful to know three damn years ago! As she flipped from page to page, all I could fixate on was my age. With each passing slide, I stuck on the *"But if you're over thirty-eight, the number of quality eggs in your body is cut in half."* It was awful, like getting taunted in school, only this time, no one could see my feelings were getting hurt and no one could hear me crying.

The next stop in this "getting to know you" afternoon appointment was to the ultrasound room—also known as the site of my first true breakdown. Yes, that's right, ladies (and the one guy whose wife made him read this), the moment Dr. Cheng did her first routine ultrasound and stuck that long magicless wand up my hoo hoo hole, I lost it. No one in the room knew what to do, including myself and my husband, who was still trying to deal with the fact that I was lying there in stirrups. I'm not entirely sure what precipitated it, but once I started, I couldn't stop.

Dr. Cheng looked at me, confused. "Why are you crying?"

I wanted to yell, *Are you serious? Did you forget about your whole thirty-eight and shriveling-up talk?* But I didn't say anything. I just wiped my eyes and waited for the time of the appointment to run out.

By the time we were back down in the building lobby, I had completely lost control of all reason. Flailing from my mouth came one illogical statement after the next, as the tears of eleven disappointing months finally freed themselves. "I'm so old. I'm fat. I'm acting like I'm pregnant, but I'm not. I haven't seen my friends. My car's too small. I feel like things with us are off. I don't feel sexy. I hate my pajamas."

Jack tried to react, but he clearly had thought I had lost my mind while he tried to keep up close behind me as my walk became an angry run. "I like your pajamas," he said, trying to make me feel better. But we both knew that it had nothing to do with my sleepwear.

It was crazy. And just when I thought the day couldn't get any worse, right smack in the middle of my breakdown came...Ella. Yes. Bouncing toward us came a friend of a friend whom I had known back in the day. She is blonde and bubbly and from the South. I actually don't even know if she is from the South. All I know is that her Southern charm wasn't quite that charming at that moment.

With the boundless energy of a four-year-old and the high-pitched voice of the Lollipop Girls, she came bouncing toward me. "Brett! Brett! How are you? What are you doing here? Do you work in this building?"

I wanted to die. The petroleum jelly was still mushing around between my legs, for God's sake, like wet feet in flip-flops when you walk home from a pedicure in the rain. "We're here to see a doctor."

Because Jack was standing next to me, she immediately jumped to the conclusion that I was pregnant. This guilty smirk came over her face like she had figured out some top-secret news. I didn't correct her. I don't know why. I knew it was only a matter of time before she would tell our mutual friend that she had seen me there, and everyone would think I was pregnant. But in that moment, I couldn't think. The day was lost.

We walked out of the building. Jack kissed me on the cheek and made his way back to work as I stood there alone on the street.

I jumped in an Uber and went to the one place that they couldn't ask any questions: Yuya Nails. All I had to do was tell them which color I wanted and then bury myself in an *US Weekly*. I went with the color "Wicked" that day. Then I put on my flip-flops and walked home—in the rain.

CHAPTER 4

MY HUSBAND'S SPERM

Is it wrong to tell you that I was completely and utterly disappointed when the results came back that my husband's sperm were healthy? I'm fully aware of how crazy that must sound. I guess a part of me was clinging to the hope that this situation wasn't all my fault—that the dried-up egg bank inside me wasn't the only guilty party in this pity parade. That ignoring my mother's plea to freeze my eggs for the past eighteen years somehow made me right. I am healthy! I was an athlete. I never did a drug in my life. (*Still sticking to it!*) I went to class. I am a CEO of a company, for God's sake. The point is, there is no logical justification for this being my fault. But it is. It's my fault. I know what you want to say. "No, it's not." But stop. Just stop.

Cheng had called us to go over Jack's results. We put the phone on speaker. "So, Jack, your sperm results are back, and everything looks great. Really great, actually. Your mobility is strong. Your count is high." I just sat there, listening on, waiting for the "but" that never came. "The quality is as high as I've seen. I don't see a problem here with any of these results."

I could hear the love affair they were having from across the phone lines. I think the only thing left for her to say was, "It was just so perfect that I took a sampling of it and put it in a locket that I will wear around my neck for always." I looked over at my husband, who I'm sure couldn't have been more thrilled to keep talking about it. I just sat there like the redheaded stepchild. All I was hearing was, "It's you. It's you. It's you," as if everyone in the room was pointing at me. All right, I get it! His sperm are perfect, and I'm an asshole. Can we get on to the next topic already?

As the results from the initial testing started to come back. Cheng could find no glaring reason why we were having trouble. She put us in a category called "unexplained." At the time, I took that as a victory and immediately started to tell myself that I didn't belong there. That I was the exception. That I would be pregnant in no time and back to the island with everyone else where I belonged, back to my normal life.

We went for a test that cleans out your fallopian tubes looking for a blockage. Some people get pregnant right after that procedure because sometimes mucus naturally blocks the sperm from having a clear path through. It clears the way, basically. I was determined that this would work for me. For us. Unfortunately, it didn't, and two weeks later we found ourselves back in Cheng's office to discuss our options.

I kept telling myself: I am not supposed to be here. I want to get back to the place where people have sex and get pregnant—where the only stress in our lives is what cute way I am going to tell my husband the good news. Maybe a T-shirt with "You're going to be a dad" on it. Put little infant shoes by the door. Leave the pee stick on his plate at dinner. We're pregnant; eat up. You'll probably have a yeast infection in your mouth, but at least we are having a baby.

I think every woman after a certain age fears being one of those "with problems" having children. You never think it will be you. I definitely didn't think it would be me. That's why when Cheng said we were going to try an IUI, I knew it would work.

An intrauterine insemination, or IUI, is essentially a turkey baster that they shove up your vagina with your partner's sperm in it. You take hormone pills to increase the amount of eggs you drop in a cycle, and then at the right time, as you are about to ovulate, they inject the sperm into you and hope that, because you have produced one or two more eggs than normal, the procedure will increase the chances of fertilization. Seems simple enough. It's just for those girls who need, you know, a little boost. I knew this would work for me.

The procedure also sometimes causes multiple eggs to fertilize. Twins! How fun would that be? Not only was this going to work, but I was going to have twins. A boy and a girl. They were going to be so close, just like my brother and me. They would be the reason I went through this whole ordeal. So, what if they weren't the first grandchildren anymore? They were "the twins," and everyone would be obsessed with them and wouldn't be able to wait for them to arrive at holidays. Their little outfits would be so cute, and they would be perfectly disheveled. I was so excited. This was sure to be the end of my journey.

After I got my period that month, Cheng put me on Clomid. It is a drug that signals your brain to send a message to the ovaries to release multiple eggs. I was to take that for five days, and then I was going to go in for an ultrasound to see how many eggs were ready to drop. The goal was two or three. Any more than that would be too dangerous for the procedure because then you could end up with quintuplets.

I took that Clomid pill religiously at the same time every day, feeling like the timing could play a role. I was desperate for any advantage I could offer myself. The biggest side effect was that it made my hormones so crazy that I could barely control my moods. But I had to stay focused and roll with it the best I could.

It wasn't just the pill though. I ate healthy and stopped drinking. I barely left my apartment other than to go to work. I wanted to do everything I could to improve our chances. I was focused. That's what good mothers do. They sacrifice. I had it in me, and I was going to beat this losing streak.

We went in on the fifth day for the ultrasound and blood work. FYI, they take blood work every time you walk into the office. Even if you come because you forgot your phone or something. The nurses, they'll find you, and they'll get ya. Their technique was about as graceful as a Greek butcher on Easter. Buy long-sleeved shirts. A lot of them. I'll leave it at that.

We had a lot riding on the result of this ultrasound. Four or more eggs could mean another lost month, which is pretty much the worst outcome at this point. I already counted the number of months we had to have this kid so that my baby would be in the same grade as my twin brother's baby. My cousins and I were so close growing up. My baby and Vince's baby had to be the same age. They just had to! If not, it would ruin a crucial tradition in our family. I didn't want my kid to be the youngest one—the one who never had a cousin counterpart and your aunt would beg you to let tag along. We had time. But not much.

We walked into the ultrasound room. The air was cooler, and only a small chink of light came in through the window. The room was small, and the ultrasound machine was stationed right smack in the middle of it. There was no way to avoid it. I gulped as I noticed the wires of all different colors and thicknesses coming out of the back—sending the information back and forth to where it needed to go.

Everyone was doing their jobs to get ready. Cheng was putting on her gloves, and the nurse was prepping the computer next to her. Jack took up his awkward position in the corner.

The nurse asked me to remove my underwear. I put my hands up my dress to grab them, and my heart sank. I could feel it—the frayed edge of that one pair of underwear that should never leave the recesses of my drawer. I must have grabbed them during the morning frenzy of getting ready. You know the pair. The one you got in your Christmas stocking in 1998 with holiday "Tic Tac Ho" on them in red and green sparkles. Would it have killed me to wear a cute pair of underwear today? What was I thinking?

What a disaster. I dragged them down my legs quickly so that no one would see. Just when I was three inches to freedom, the thong part got caught on my pinky toe. The toe that never had a function until this very moment was now determined to not release this underwear from complete exposure. Everyone turned around to see what was going on. They pretended to not be paying attention, but I know they saw. I felt them judging.

This underwear was so stretched out that there is no logical reason that it should get caught on anything. I'm surprised it even stayed on me at all. It defied gravity. I stood there tugging for dear life as they all looked on—the love of my life, Cheng, the Greek butcher—all patiently waiting for me to lie back on the table. With one desperate tug, they came free—a Christmas fucking miracle. I shoved the underwear into my shoe and jumped up on the table. Right then and there, I made a promise to my future daughter: I will only be getting her sexy underwear for her stocking. Even when she's twelve. Just in case.

As I lay down, my nerves were going crazy. My stomach was turning. Have you ever tried to hold in a poop when your legs are spread apart on stirrups? Let's just say my Facebook status that day should've read, "It's complicated."

Dr. Cheng started making small talk, but my eye was on the prize. I needed to know what was swimming around in there. She put Petroleum Jelly on the wand and slowly put it in. She moved it around.

Jack and I were glued to the screen. She started with the left side. I felt the pressure of her moving it inside me. She didn't speak. I'm no doctor, but it was pretty obvious she wasn't finding anything to see. This went on for what felt like minutes but was probably only ten seconds or so.

"Okay, nothing on that side," she said.

My heart dropped. No eggs? That wasn't an option I had considered. Did I even have ovaries? What was she seeing? She then moved the wand to the other side. I felt the pressure move away from one side of my body to the other. At this point, I felt my insides push pause. I was fixated on the screen, watching in silence, but ready to scream on the inside.

"Oh, there we go. This side seems awake. There's one." She paused and kept probing. I felt the pressure of her moving the wand aggressively around. "There's two..." Yes! Yes! We were in the game! I sat up a little in order to get a closer view of the screen. "Three..." Oh man! We had three! WE HAD THREE! Oh wait, we can't have four. Cheng had to stop at three. I wanted to grab that wand out of her hand and smash it on the floor before she could find any more.

She kept investigating as if she was determined to find the fourth. I then felt the wand slowly slip from my vagina, and Dr. Cheng tapped me on the knee. "All right, we have three."

I was so happy I could've run down Seventh Avenue without putting my underwear back on! Holiday Tic Tac Ho underwear for everyone next year!

We played it cool until everyone left the room. Once the door closed, my husband and I grabbed each other tightly, and I started to cry. We had done it. This was the start of our family.

We went back downtown with huge smiles on our faces. We went to our favorite brunch spot, Bubby's, and ordered pancakes. I knew we would talk about this for years to come. We had one week and then we would go in for the procedure. I couldn't wait. I was watching my dreams unfold before my eyes.

Forty-eight hours before the scheduled IUI, I had to take what's called a "trigger shot" to initiate ovulation. That way, the doctors can control exactly when I ovulate. Once I start to ovulate, then they implant the sperm into my uterus and hope that as the egg drops, it can marry up with the sperm at the perfect time, increasing the chances of it fertilizing.

This was my first official injection that didn't take place in a doctor's office. I had to take it at home. I was panicked, even though the needle was tiny. I left it in the middle of my kitchen counter for a week. We had a stare-off every day. It owned me. It was all I could think about. The doctor called and said to take it at eight. We woke up early, and Jack prepped the shot. Jack is a "read the fine print" type of guy. After reading the twenty-two-inch-long paper directions, we were ready. He knew everything there was to know about the shot, right down to where it was manufactured. I think he even read the side that was in Chinese. He took off the cap. Tapped it a few times to get the air bubbles out and then looked over at me. I must have looked like the last puppy to be sold in the litter, crunched alone in the corner of the cage. I had somehow managed to lodge myself in between the chair and the table.

Jack just smirked. "All right, kiddo, let's do this." He brought the needle toward me. He took a three-inch start and then jammed it into my stomach. I jumped as if it hurt, but it surprisingly didn't. Like at all. I wish I had a book like this to tell me that. *(You're welcome!)* I had been shitting my pants all week over this, and as it turned out, the anticipation was the worst part. No matter what, it was over, and I was pumped. I jumped in my car and headed down to Philly, where I had a client meeting.

I started to mull over what happened as I drove down the Turnpike. I was so relieved the shot was over. I remembered reading that the trigger shot was to be taken forty-eight hours before the IUI. So that would bring me to Thursday. Wait, Thursday? My IUI was Friday. As I drew up my fingers to count on my hand two days from now, I confirmed forty-eight hours would be Thursday! What had I done? Was I supposed to take the shot in the p.m.? No one told me p.m. Or did they? Did I just assume a.m.? Did I ruin it? The medicine was already well on its way inside of me. Did we do all of this for nothing?

I called the doctor, but all I could get was the receptionist. She took down my question as if I was a crazy psycho GOMO that she was sick of dealing with, giving me the not-so-subtle impression that my question wasn't a valid one.

A nurse came on the line. She said we "should" be okay. SHOULD? What does that mean?! Were they taking me seriously? We couldn't lose another month. We just couldn't! Especially for silly mistakes.

Between my anxiety and the Clomid, I was on the express train to crazy town. I had no choice but to trust her and wait. Guilt poured over me like hot wax. This was so typical of me to screw up a detail like this. Do I even tell Jack? Would he be mad? My life was closing in on me.

I just kept driving. I had no choice but to trust the nurse and wait.

CHAPTER 5

MY BASTER ON THE SIDE

It was the Friday of Easter weekend. The sun was shining. We were heading down to the shore that night to my parents' beach house with my entire family for the holiday. Just three letters stood between us and the relaxing weekend we were so looking forward to: I. U. I. Jack and I woke up that morning ready to attack the day. Jack had to go about an hour before me to do his "thing." And when I say his "thing," I mean, whack off in a weird little masturbation room, into a little clear jar, and hand it to a nurse who either magically appeared as soon as he was finished, or worse, would be standing outside the door the entire time. The procedure was actually hysterical. Well, it was hysterical if you were me. But for him it was mortifying. I didn't really see what the big deal was. He was like a celebrity in there. You know, him and his perfect sperm and all. I wanted to help the cause, though. He was going to fertilize our twins! It had to be good!

After Jack left for the doctor's office, I quickly went to my closet. My plan was to put on some lingerie, take some sexy pictures and send them to him by the time he made it to the "good time room." So at least I was somehow with him. Deep in the back of my closet was a box filled with lingerie. I wish I could say that this was a box that guys dream women had, with leather whips and furry undies in it. But not this one. Mine had a few sexy pieces of lingerie, but man, did you have to dig to find them.

I started to look through the box. I pulled out a random vibrator in the shape of the Eiffel Tower that my cousin brought me back from Europe as a joke years ago. I found a bra with Jack's head ironed on it, a gift from one of my bridesmaids—a few silk robes that were given to me by an aunt of some sort. I kept digging. I needed something next level. Something he hadn't seen in a while. Not just my go-to. And then I saw it, peeking out from the corner of the box. Valentine's Day, 2015. The thigh highs and garter were perfect. They were sure to get his mind exactly where it needed to be.

I didn't have unlimited time. It would probably take Jack twenty minutes to get uptown to Cheng's office. I pulled the stockings up fast. Not sure if you have ever tried to put thigh-high stockings on, but there is no such thing as putting them on quickly. I was bouncing around, trying to get them up. When I pulled them to their maximum length and they fell right above my knee, I knew something was wrong and I had to start over. The nylons looked more like a tourniquet than a sexy thigh-high! At this point I hadn't even brushed my teeth yet. Sweat was gathering on my upper lip, and my armpits were starting to get ripe. I attached the tights to the little clips on the top of the underwear. I'm sure this was not like the slow-motion sexy way the Victoria's Secret models do it before a shoot.

I went for the bra. Where the hell was the bra! Oh Jesus. I started chucking things all over the place. I found a bustier that could work. I strapped it on with one fastener, bypassing the eighteen little clips in the back. I grabbed my phone and raced toward the mirror.

What I saw in the reflection was not really what I had in mind. It looked like a cross between Cher from 1970 and Shrek from 2001. The thigh-highs were so tight that my upper thigh fat was pouring over the tops. The loose skin on my belly was somehow protruding out of the bottom of the bustier. I didn't have time to fuss. It was time to suck in and start snapping.

I set the timer and placed the phone against the wall so it could stand up on its own. I pushed the button and then ran to get into my sexy position. I changed my face a few times in the five seconds I had and then I heard the snap. I ran to the camera to see what it looked like. Bam, a picture of my dresser and ceiling.

I didn't realize being sexy would be so tough. The racing back and forth went on for a few tries. Some showed too much fat while others captured my horrible attempts at making a sexy face. I mean, what was that? It looked like I was angry. And possessed. And being held hostage by Russian porn traffickers. I finally realized my face wouldn't be making any magic in that little room for Jack, so I snapped a few from behind and pushed send. I got the photo I needed.

After my Playboy interlude, I jumped in an Uber to meet Jack at the doctor's office. The traffic was a little heavier than usual. I remember watching all the women walking to work and wondering if they had kids. It's funny how you can suddenly become so aware of what you don't want to see on a city street. New York is tough on you like that. When you are single, you see couples holding hands and laughing. When you are lonely, you see groups of friends laughing and busting each other's chops. And when you are trying to have a baby, you see mothers and their kids—everywhere. Why was it so easy for them? I tried to look away, but the image was still so vivid in my mind.

The Uber pulled up, and I got out of the car and made my way up to the office. It was my turn, and it was going to be a good day. When I walked into the waiting room, I saw Jack sitting there. He had this guilty smile on his face, which made me realize he had gotten my pictures. He greeted me with a big hug. When he pressed up against me, I could feel the sweat on his chest from through his shirt. New territory for all of us, I guess.

We walked into the ultrasound room. I immediately noticed all the tools on the counter. All lined up for me. It could've been a pile of teddy bears, and it would've freaked me out. But I was choosing to be brave. Kids with life-threatening diseases face far worse every day. I could certainly get through this.

I started to undress. Before I had left that morning, I made sure to put on a nice lacy pair of underwear. I didn't want a repeat of the Tic Tac Ho incident of two weeks ago. I had to show Cheng that I had a little sass in me. I wanted Jack to be proud. I wanted the nurse to silently think to herself, *Wow, this girl must be something else.* This was my chance to regain my street credit.

I went up my skirt and slowly pulled my underwear down. This time nobody noticed. I pulled them up again really quickly and then tried again. Nothing. I even did a fake jump to get their attention, but no one turned. Oh, now suddenly they had more important things to do than staring at me remove my underwear? I sighed as I let them linger on my shoe as a last-ditch effort to gain their attention, but no one cared. I jumped up on the table and waited. Cheng wasn't there yet, so there was still hope.

I lay there while the nurse bustled about in the silence of the room. Jack, who usually stays a safe distance away from the stirrups, pushed his chair closer to me and grabbed my hand. He looked at me with hope in his eyes. It was warm and kind. I smiled back. I think it was his attempt to make this special for us. We might not be able to recall that romantic night that our kids were conceived. But we were going to have this.

The door opened, and someone walked in. I saw sneakers. I looked up toward the face. Who was this? Where was Cheng? Where were her trendy shoes and her serious composure? In walked "Tammi." I don't think she even introduced herself as *Dr.* Tammi. Just Tammi. She started to put her gloves on casually as if she was about to make a salami sandwich at the local Subway. I warily asked, "Where is Dr. Cheng?"

Tammi replied in a bouncy yet blunt voice, "Oh, she's not in today."

Not in today? What could be more important than the fertilization of my twins? She needed to be here! For me! For the twins! For the God-damned lacy underwear! I'm sure Tammi has done these hundreds of times, right? I mean, I think so. How could we possibly know? She had yoga pants on for God's sake! I took a deep breath and tried to relax.

Tammi sat down and grabbed her instruments. There was a long syringe that had a vial next to it. I looked at it closely, making sure there were no secret needles anywhere, but it seemed like the coast was clear. Jack leaned in closer, knowing that we were about to get started. "Are you scared?" he asked.

The question caught me off guard. It never crossed my mind to be scared. Maybe I was. Maybe I wasn't. I didn't know what I was feeling. All I knew was that I needed this to work. "I'm just ready," I answered back.

The "doctor" rolled her chair over and began. She put one instrument inside me and started to push. I felt more pain than I thought I would, but at least I knew she was helping me make my baby. I held Jack's hand tighter.

Just when I thought the pain was about to get worse, the procedure was done. I was informed that I had to lie there for twenty minutes and then I could go on my way. We were to return in three weeks to take a pregnancy blood test to see if it worked.

Tammi and the nurse started to head toward the door. Right before Tammi exited the room, she peeked back in and said, "Don't forget to have sex tonight and tomorrow."

Wait, what? Sex? Cheng never told us that! Was this something Tammi and her Pilates friends made up just to mess with us? Was this woman even part of the practice? Maybe she saw the underwear and assumed. Damn underwear screwed me again. She closed the door behind her.

Jack and I sat in the silent vacuum. Meditating on our own thoughts. I became aware of a weird heaviness in the air. "How do you feel?" Jack asked, breaking the silence.

"I feel good. I think. Could this really be it?"

He held my hand harder. "I can't believe it's all happening inside of you right now. Can you feel it?"

"Not really. But I feel it in my gut. I know this is going to work for us."

Jack kept smiling at me and stroking the top of my head. This could be the time we remembered as the one that we became a true family. It felt intimate. It felt hopeful. Even amidst all the heaviness surrounding us. This was our ticket out of here.

Jack helped me down from the table. He stood close as I got dressed just in case I lost my footing. My body was shaking as I walked slowly toward the door, not knowing how to soak in what had just happened. I felt alone even with Jack close beside me. All our hopes were resting on me and no one else. We were holding hands, but we were walking in two separate worlds.

As I headed down the hall toward the waiting room, I saw a face walking toward us that looked vaguely familiar. As I got closer, I realized that we had gone to the same college. She was in my sorority, but I really didn't know her well. I might have said ten words to her in my entire four years there. Maybe our circle of friends never crossed. Maybe we had nothing in common back then. Yet our eyes met, and it felt familiar and warm. We gravitated toward each other. She grabbed me, and we hugged. We didn't even exchange words. She started to cry in my arms. I held her as tight as I could. I felt tears start to gather in the corners of my eyes. It all hit me in that moment. She wasn't alone. And neither was I.

Jack pulled the car up to the front of the building, and I slowly climbed in, careful not to disturb the precious cargo inside me. It was time to head down to the Jersey Shore for Easter weekend, where all my cousins, aunts, and uncles would be waiting—a much-needed break from reality. It was time to put all the emotions of the day behind us.

I come from a huge Italian family. We literally travel in herds—big, loud, amazing herds where everyone has his or her role. Apart, we are just a group of random dysfunctional people with inappropriate humor, but together, we are a perfectly oiled machine and the chemistry is nothing short of magic—chaotic magic, but magic still. I knew if I could make it down to the shore house, all the emotions of today would get lost in fart jokes and sarcasm and the world would start feeling normal again. I didn't know how to process all the emotions I was feeling. But at least the first step was over.

With each mile Jack and I drove, we shed more and more stress. We knew everyone else had already been down there all day. We listened to music on the radio and slowly settled into a good place. Though the Clomid was still ripe in my system, I was starting to get my center of balance back. I was ready to put this day behind me.

My phone started buzzing, and I saw it was my mom. I thought she was calling to see where we were or to ask us to pick up something along the way. But when I picked up, she asked, "What should we do? Uncle Jimmy is here, but he may be leaving soon."

I had no idea what she was worried about. Timing? Where we would sleep? Dinner? I answered, "Well, that's okay. He can stay in our room."

She replied, "No, he's leaving. Should we wait?"

Wait for what? What was she talking about?

"The announcement. Vince and Grace? They want to announce to everyone together about the baby."

I sat there, stunned, unaware of everything around me. Center of balance lost. Feeling like huge weights were tied to the back of my tonsils I said, "We'll be there in ten minutes."

I had completely forgotten about their announcement. Just as much as they had likely forgotten that my appointment was today. I tried to make sense of all the different feelings that were battling inside me: sadness, guilt, hurt. I didn't know which one was going to win.

"What was that about?" Jack asked.

"Nothing really, they just wanted to know where we were because

Vince and Grace are going to make the announcement about their baby."

I waited for a response from him, but it never came. I knew that everyone would be waiting for us. I could hear the shouts from blocks away "Hey! Brett! Ahh!" That's what we do. We scream and cheer when someone walks in and then you kiss. You kiss everyone. I was doomed.

When we pulled up to the beach house, Jack dropped me off and went to look for a parking spot. I walked in as I had so many times before. The familiar salty smell of the living room filled the air. I had hardly taken a step inside before catching my mother's eye, and I knew I was about to lose it. My chin started to tremble, and I felt my throat tighten up. My cheeks started to tingle right below my eyes.

I ran through the living room, saying I had to pee in an effort to bypass the kissing stage. I got to the bathroom, closed the door behind me, and burst into tears. There was nothing I could do to stop it as hard as I tried. I knew they were all waiting for me. I knew they would know I was crying. I didn't want to take away from my brother's moment, but I didn't know how to pull myself together enough to get out of the bathroom.

Finally, I took a few deep breaths, splashed some water on my face, and opened the door. My two cousins were waiting right outside for me. They must have sensed something was up. They tried to hug me, but I knew that if they did, I would lose it again. I walked back out to the living room and pretended I had to get something out of the car. I gave Jack the eye to follow me.

Once we reached the safety of the car again, I felt my body give in. Give in to the hurt that I had been fighting all day. Give in to the guilt. Give in to the embarrassment of seeing my fucking underwear in my shoe over and over again.

Jack touched my leg and watched on. It wasn't like me to get so upset. "You don't have to hold it in. Take a deep breath," he said.

I breathed in through my nose and out through my mouth in three hard pulls and pushes. I needed this pause to reset.

"This is about us now," Jack said. "Don't worry about anyone else. Tell me what you're feeling."

I didn't know how to answer him. I felt like everything we had gone through was all hitting me at once. The words floated out of my mouth—the answer to the question I didn't know the answer to hours before when he asked. "Yes, I am scared."

He grabbed the back of my head and pulled it in to his chest as I cried. I drew strength from his support. He never made me feel crazy or unjustified. He didn't try to make me feel better. He just listened. And he was there. I regained my composure after ten minutes, and I felt recharged enough to go back inside.

Grace had made up little Easter cards for everyone that were hidden inside brightly colored plastic eggs. It said, "Our little bunny will be here in October." After we were all gathered together, she had my mother hand out the eggs to everyone as if it was some group activity. Everyone opened them at the same time: "1...2...3!" I looked on as the news hit each of them one by one. The joy in their eyes. The surprise. The happiness. An announcement that I had envisioned for myself. While Grace was folding up her cute Easter cards that morning, I was getting violated by syringes and speculums. Everyone hugged them and screamed and jumped up and down. I did as well. But it was an act. I was dying inside. People glanced at me and then looked away. Did they pity me? Did they wonder when it would happen for me? Did they even care?

Vince and Grace did the same egg trick the next day when my other cousin, Frank, and his wife, Leah, came down. It was the same show all over again—like watching your own death twice. The only difference this time was that after the cheering for them ended, Frank and Leah yelled in unison: "We're pregnant too!" I was empty.

CHAPTER 6

CLOMID

What kind of fucked-up human being invented Clomid? Seriously. It had to be a lab test gone wrong. Did lab rats start crying uncontrollably and stabbing each other all at the same time, and some mad scientist thought, *Hmmm, maybe I can give this to women at their most vulnerable time and watch them self-implode.* For those of you who aren't familiar with the drug, Clomid is a hormone pill that you take for five days after your period ends. It prompts your brain to tell your ovaries to drop multiple eggs in a cycle instead of one. The problem is it makes you bat-shit crazy at the same time. This is probably why a casual walk into the shore house filled with family on Easter weekend became like a scene out of *The Exorcist*.

I consider myself a fairly rational person. But man, once you get a few of those beauties in you, you never know what will happen. That weekend wasn't the only episode. I would find myself crying in my office and in random parking lots before client meetings, blowing my nose into dry cleaning in the backseat of my car. I would literally have to analyze which piece of clothing to use.

I'd be in this hysterical, world-is-ending crying attack, and then pause to think to myself, *Maybe not this dress. I may wear it Saturday.* I often chose one of my husband's work shirts. They always felt the nicest on my nose. It's the least he could endure for having "perfect sperm."

I'd get so angry over the simplest setbacks—like emotions on crack. The smallest annoyance could set me off. Driving in the city was the worst. Didn't matter who it was: the dog walker with earphones on who didn't realize the light had changed, delivery guys on bikes in the wrong lane, delivery guys on bikes in the right lane, commuters, children, pigeons, the sun, anything. I literally had to invent a game with myself that when I got really angry, I would put my hand below the window line, so no one else could see, and flick off whoever I was mad at. I would give them the finger like a ten-year-old in the back of a bus on a class trip. They couldn't see it. I kept it real low. You know, kept it classy. The gesture wasn't meant for them anyway. I was doing it for me.

If you have to take Clomid, my only advice is to embrace it. Don't fight it. Know that crazy is coming and own it. Know it is not really you. Warn your husband. Warn your friends. Warn the women and children in your neighborhood. You know what? Warn everyone: Even the guy that makes your coffee at Starbucks every morning. "I said SKIM MILK!"

"It is skim milk, miss."

"Oh, okay. Well, just making sure you knew. *I'm watching you.*"

Husbands out there, now may be a good time to incorporate a

nice foot massage into your at-home routine. Clean the dishes. Wear a helmet. You know, the basics. Your sweet blushing bride will be back soon. Not too soon, but soon.

CHAPTER 7

LONDON BRIDGE IS FALLING DOWN

For the next two weeks, I tried to stay as busy as possible to keep my mind off whether the IUI had worked. The weekend before we were to get the result, we attended my cousin Marla's wedding in London. The wedding was that Saturday. We were due to fly back Sunday night in time for our Monday morning appointment in New York.

Marla was not merely my cousin; she was my best friend. I had spent my entire life idolizing her. She was like a sister to me. I will never forget feeling so badly that I couldn't party it up for her at the wedding. But my eye was on the prize, and I had to stay focused. I was essentially pregnant, so I had to be on my best behavior. No drinks. No coffee. No late nights. I'm not going to say it didn't take a little bit away from the weekend for me, but I had no choice. We had lost so many months already, what was one more? I had the blood pregnancy test at Cheng's office set for that Monday after we got back. I had snuck a pregnancy test in my toiletry bag just in case. I knew that this was against the rules, but I had to bring it.

On the morning after the wedding, I woke up around six o'clock and couldn't fall back asleep. I tried to distract myself with the joyous events of the night before, but all I could think about was that test. I had started to feel some cramping at the wedding. Could that be what my best friend Dr. Google calls "implantation cramping?" I needed to know. Were my efforts of the week paying off?

This was the perfect time. My husband was still passed out next to me. It was my only opportunity. I snuck into the bathroom and slowly closed the door, careful not to wake him up. I grabbed the pregnancy test out of my bag and started to tear it open, trying not to make a sound. With no scissors in sight, I bit and tried to tear the packaging open. The plastic wasn't budging. My hands were clammy and starting to shake.

I gave the package one huge tear, the seams burst open, and the test went flying. With my bladder about to explode, I crab-walked over to where it landed, grabbed it, and headed back to the toilet. I placed the test between my legs. I looked down to make sure I was peeing on the stick and then I saw it. A bright red glob. I had literally gotten my period on the pregnancy test.

I heard Jack stirring in the other room. "Honey, are you okay?"

"I'm fine," which was usually code word for "I'm indisposed." But I wasn't indisposed. I was sitting there in disbelief. I looked down at the stick again and the words "not pregnant" started to appear. I didn't cry. I didn't do anything. I just sat there trying to figure out what to do next. Do I tell Jack? Do I let him enjoy that feeling of hope for another few hours?

I went back in the room and got into bed. He lifted his head and saw my face. He opened up the blankets as if to invite me in. He pulled me in close to him. He already knew.

A month later, the second IUI didn't work either. The future started to look dark. Really dark. I was officially in the "one of those girls with problems" club. I felt like a complete and utter failure. For the first time in my life, I had a problem that I could not fix. I felt lost in my own skin and a stranger to people I used to find comfort in. Positive thoughts fled my body in a mass exodus. And just when I thought I couldn't feel any lower, I realized where we were headed: in vitro fertilization. IVF.

CHAPTER 8

NEEDLING

I'll never forget the night the bag of drugs showed up at our apartment. We had been out drinking on one of those rare nights when we had forgotten what was going on. Jack and I were walking arm in arm as I took the last ten steps that my feet could handle in my tall boots. "You are so right. These boots were totally worth it," Jack joked sarcastically as he helped me limp inside with my throbbing feet.

"It's your fault. You fell in love with me at five-foot-six, not five-foot-two. What do you want me to do?" I giggled.

As we approached the front desk, the doorman said we had a package. We were thrilled—the type of thrilled you used to get when your mom sent you a care package at college. Neither of us remembered ordering anything. The doorman came out with a box so huge that you could barely see him. Our faces lit up. Was it a late wedding gift? Was it a case of fresh oranges from Florida? Was it something we've never even heard of before? The possibilities were endless! We lugged it upstairs with the excitement of two six-year-olds on Christmas morning.

The second we walked into the apartment, I ran toward the knife block. I grabbed the first steak knife I could lay my hand on and headed for the box. Jack yelled to me, "Use the scissors! You know how many germs are on those boxes!"

"It's fine. I'm in manufacturing. This is better."

"All good, I love plastic wrap in my steak."

"Shush, I'm concentrating."

I slowly slid the knife through the top. I didn't want to rip the fragile gift that was sure to be waiting inside. We opened the lid and found the usual little foam inserts. I swiped them out of the way without a second thought. I could see the tip of something. I lifted the bag out of the box, and the foam inserts spilled every-where. I looked inside. There it was: the largest Ziploc bag that I had ever seen, filled with medicines and vials. Syringe after syringe, the lineup kept going. The pain had left my feet and lodged itself deep into my stomach. Ready or not, the journey had officially begun.

I grabbed the bag, raised it over my head, and yelled, "Game on, bitches!"

The silence was broken, and we laughed. Jack put the music on loud. We shoved the boxes to the side and jumped around like two drunken idiots. Naïve maybe, but it was thrilling—thrilling to be the couple that was going to laugh our way through this ordeal, empowering to be the woman who would not let this break her.

We took pictures of the ridiculous number of drugs lined up like soldiers ready for battle on our counter and sent it to some of our friends. It was not the road we chose to go down, but it was ours. We would do what we needed to do—retrieve as many eggs as we could and then move on with our lives. This was it. I was almost excited. I had this inner strength inside me. I was ready. It was game day, and I was ready to play. Prick me, prod me. Do what you need to do. I was going to look back on all of this and be proud of myself. Proud of us for staying strong. Proud of us for doing what we needed to do for our family.

Not only was this process going to help us make our baby, but we would be able to bank eggs for our future children. Whatever the number was, fifteen, twenty eggs! I could make a whole village after this! It made so much sense. Two weeks of shots, that's all I had to get through and then this would be past us. We had this. I had this.

When I say, "I had this," I should've mentioned one minor problem. I. Hate. Needles. I mean, like, really hate needles. I was the kid in the doctor's office who would hide in the corner kicking and screaming on vaccination day. So, when one week later we started the injections, you can imagine how freaked out I was.

Weeks back when we were at Cheng's office, we had a training session with a nurse on how to use the shots and the various needles and what they all did. Because, of course, they are all completely different. At the time, we had almost completed our second IUI. I was so convinced it was going to work that I wasn't paying attention to the training because that wasn't us. We weren't IVF people. "Those people."

I remember joking about it in the office, like laughing in class. But shit got real when it was go time, and we realized we had retained absolutely nothing. I actually felt like I knew less about the shots after that session.

The idea of the shots was terrifying to me. It wasn't just the shots, though. It was all of the paraphernalia, too: the big sharps container to dispose of the syringes, the various sizes of needles sprawled all over the table. I have had sex with my husband on this table, for God's sake, and now it looked like an emergency room filled with needles and alcohol wipes.

Jack read all the material like a good banker does. And I just sat there—like a good printer does.

"Okay," Jack said, "so we have to make sure the shot is a few inches to the side of the belly button. Hold on, let me check on something." As he clicked away on his phone. "It's fine," I said, "they just mean somewhere in this area." As I pointed to the bottom of my stomach. "It doesn't have to be exact."

"Well, I'm pretty sure it does have to be exact. Give me a second. Let me just look on YouTube."

As he searched, all these videos came up. Cute women in yoga pants and pigtails stabbing themselves with needles. Sexy, brave, and more than anything else, calm. *Seriously?* Who made these videos? Obviously not a woman. Where was the girl code in that?

My husband was looking at these amazing stomachs on these videos, and now I was going to have to lift my shirt to expose a pasty white abdomen that hasn't seen a gym in a year. Okay, two years. (Be nice to me. I'm in IVF!) That's all I need in my fragile state—to walk in and see my husband ogling the girl in the IVF video.

"You were totally checking out the girl in that video!"

"I was not!"

"You keep going back to her!"

"She's just extra...thorough."

"And an extra bra size up."

"It has nothing to do with that," he said as he smiled.

"Yeah right." I gave his shoulder a nudge as he laughed.

"Okay, come on, get back to business here."

He was obviously nervous to get it right. So was I, but I tried to keep a brave face. I was going to be the girl who was positive and somehow made this fun. That is who I am and who I wanted to be. So, I put my hair in pigtails and "woman-ed" up.

The regimen was one shot of Follistim in the morning and a shot of Lupron and Menopur at night. The Follistim and Menopur help to stimulate the development and growth of multiple eggs within the ovaries. The Lupron keeps you from ovulating so the eggs can grow without the body naturally releasing them.

Once we nailed down the spot, Jack grabbed my stomach. "I'm going to count to three. You ready?"

"Absolutely not."

"Come on. I'll do it quickly."

"Okay, do it fast. Actually, maybe do it slow. Think it's better slow?"

"You've got this. One...two...three." And in it went. He slowly pushed the meds in and then pulled out the needle. "Done. You okay?"

"That wasn't so bad," I said, convincing myself as well. "Wow, we did it." A little drop of blood seeped out from where he put the injection in. He put a tissue over it. "First shot done!" he exclaimed as he put his hands in the air.

We hugged each other and tried to laugh, but the last hour had completely exhausted us. We both let out a huge sigh of relief. "Only 39 more to go!" I laughed.

Jack got up early each morning and rushed home at night to give me every single injection for the next two weeks. I won't say getting poked so often was easy, but it wasn't the worst thing either. The thought was worse than the prick. It just gave me the willies.

Every. Single. Time. I would wake up in the middle of the night and cringe thinking about it. Waiting in anticipation for seven o' clock. The timing of these shots was very important. They had to be ten hours apart from each other. They say that the more consistent you are with the timing, the better. But who knows? What I've come to learn is that no one really knows anything for sure.

We did learn that it was tough to plan it early enough in the morning to still get to work on time and late enough to be back in time at the end of the day. Seems simple enough, but the daily ritual was pretty disruptive. Even client dinners had to go on hold because of the timing of these shots. But it was our priority. We just had to make it through two weeks, and we'd be back in the game with everyone else.

After a few days, we had the routine down. Jack would prepare the concoction. I would wait. He would carefully choose the exact spot on my stomach to inject. He would swab the area profusely. Count to three and poke me—directly outside the swabbed area. I didn't have the heart to tell him that he was missing it. He was putting so much heart into it. I always thought it was sweet, though, that he was there with me. It made me feel he was taking care of me and that we were truly in this together. He held up his end, to the point that I didn't have to think about it.

I'm very absent minded. I'm more of a Cliff's Notes kind of girl. Oftentimes we would have a situation where I forgot to order a med that we needed, or I measured something wrong. I'd end up in the only same-day pharmacy that existed for fertility drugs on the uppermost tip of Manhattan in a panic. These minor mishaps made me so frustrated with myself every time. You think that you are going to ruin everything. In my defense, the doctors leave an awful lot of responsibility to the patient. I guess everyone figures out how to make the regimen work, but still, it's frightening.

Note to IVF Peeps: Check your drugs! Don't trust the process. Make sure you have everything you need because the running-out shit sneaks up on you. There's nothing worse than realizing you have to take a drug that you don't have. I'll save you from that panic and the silent argument you are sure to have with your husband while you both try to figure out who was to blame for this. Pay attention. Save your cycle. *Save your marriage.*

After a few days of injections, I was scheduled to see Cheng for bloodwork and an ultrasound. I was feeling pretty good. You know, besides the fact that I was starting and ending my days with several needles to the abdomen. That was the weirdest part. Going to work every day knowing that this was going on. Knowing that no one knew how your morning started or the private struggle you were having. It made me realize that you never know what someone is carrying on their shoulders every day. It's something I never really thought about before. You assume everyone came from a happy morning eating pancakes, but unfortunately that's not the case. A smile can go a long way. We should all do it more. A part of me enjoyed the escape of being at work. It kept me distracted even though it was hard to concentrate on anything else.

Jack offered to come with me when it came time to check in with Cheng, as he did with every other appointment, but I told him it was no big deal. They were only going to take bloodwork and do an ultrasound, and then I would be on my way. There was no need for both of us to ruin our mornings at work.

I walked into Cheng's reception room, and they called me in right away for bloodwork. I was feeling pretty good. At the core of all of this was the start of our family, and I tried not to lose sight of the purpose. I did mention how much I hate the bloodwork, yes? I would always try to sweet-talk the nurse before she stuck the needle in so she would go easy on me.

After the bloodwork came the ultrasound. I wasn't really sure what they were checking for, but I assumed they wanted to make sure the drugs were working. It was part of the routine.

I was shown into a different room than I had used before. It smelled like plastic, as if they had just started using it. I lowered my underwear into my shoe and jumped up onto the table. I noticed that a light above the table had no bulb in it. I fixated on that as I waited.

Cheng came in. "Good morning. Let's see what we've got here." For the first time, she mentioned a word that would become the focus of the future as I knew it: follicles.

Cheng took her little wand out and placed it inside me. She moved it around and started measuring what she was calling follicles. I had no idea what she meant, but I listened and observed, not too fazed by it. Oddly, I was feeling more curious about the bulb-less light above my head. She measured these follicles and then called out the measurements to the nurse. She counted six.

I had never heard the word follicle before. "What do those numbers mean?" I asked.

"It means you have six eggs growing."

I wasn't sure how to react. *Six?* I thought I was supposed to get like twenty! In every story I had ever heard women got fifteen, twenty, even thirty! But six? A bout of tears was coming on hard and fast. I felt it.

"It's still early and there could be some sleepers that mature late. We will keep checking every few days."

Once Cheng left the room, I broke down crying. I didn't understand. Could this be right? Was this measly result what they thought would happen? Were all the shots even working? I didn't realize they could tell so early.

I tried to calm myself down. I didn't have the energy to call Jack yet. I felt dizzy and heavy—like the walls were closing in on me with every step as I walked out of that awful room. I somehow made it to the lobby. I was one foot away from the door when the receptionist stopped me and said, "You need to pay."

I was so frazzled. As I gave her my credit card, she explained that she had to charge for the entire cycle. Like right now. She grabbed my card before I could even think what she meant and charged the full amount. $22,000. I thought I was inside a nightmare. I was unable to speak, to voice all the questions I would have normally asked. I just needed to escape that place. My credit card somehow went through. I signed the slip and walked out. I must have looked like a ghost.

I flopped down into my car and called Jack. He soaked in the news as he always does and then tried to comfort me. "It's still early, sweetness. Who knows what will happen? We have six eggs, and that's better than none. And don't forget the possible sleepers."

In a daze, I managed to drive through the Lincoln Tunnel and out into Jersey. I pulled off at the first rest stop I could find. I found a parking spot isolated from the other cars and just sat there. Staring into nothing. Unable to comprehend what I was feeling.

Finally, I called my mother. She asked a lot of questions—none of which I knew the answers to. We both tried to make sense of the disappointing results. We needed to stay positive. My mom tried to comfort me, but nothing felt right. I didn't even know what I wanted to hear. It just hurt, and there wasn't really anything anyone could say.

"It'll all work out."

"Stay positive."

"Let's see what happens."

They all felt like empty words. After I started to feel somewhat normal again, I began to drive to work. I had to get through the day. I had to put on a strong face. Deals had to be done, and problems had to be solved. There was no time for these tears. I had to stay positive. I had this. I think.

A dark thought lurked in the back of my mind. I had to go back in three days. That's how these cycles go. Once you start the hormone treatments, they test you every few days to see how the follicles are progressing. Via some thorough Google searching of what a follicle actually is, I informed myself, no thanks to my doctor.

In an ultrasound, they can't see eggs, but they can see follicles. Follicles house the eggs. If an egg grows and starts to mature, the follicle will grow. Counting follicles gives the doctors an idea as to how many eggs they may be retrieving and how mature they are. They retrieve everything regardless, but the procedure is a gauge to measure the sizes so they know when it's time for retrieval. They want the follicles to grow larger than fifteen centimeters, if not twenty.

All of these facts fell into the category of things MY DOCTOR SHOULD'VE TOLD ME WHEN WE STARTED! Maybe a "lay of the land" chat would've helped ease the blow. You know, a little "what to expect when you're *not* expecting." Maybe they did, and we just didn't pay attention. At this point, I had no idea about anything, and I was starting to lose traction.

By the time of my next appointment, I had my emotions back in check. I went in hoping that more follicles had matured. During those three days, I took my meds perfectly and knew that we were bound to have some follicles that were late bloomers. I reminded myself that I didn't have any health issues. I was barely even an IVF patient. Also, like the doctor said, I had to be patient and give the immature eggs time to grow. Either way, I made peace with my six. No matter what, I had six, and I was going to will these little guys to grow big and strong.

Three days later, I found myself back on the table again. With all her condescending Zen, in walked "Dr." Tammi. Ugh. Okay, it was fine. She had a degree. She had patients of her own. I just needed to know the number of eggs.

Tammi put the wand in and started to move it around. She spewed out all kinds of numbers. I tried to follow, but the tension was unbearable. "One at fifteen"..."one at twelve"..."Here are two less than ten." She finally pulled out the wand.

I'm no math whiz, but I could've sworn she only counted four. "Excuse me, Doctor—oh, I'm sorry, I mean Tammi, how many did you say you saw?"

"I see four growing."

Four? Where were the other two? Where were the sleepers I was promised? I didn't know having fewer was an option. Suddenly six sounded like a great number. I'm sorry I was sad at six. I'll take six back! I want six back!

Tammi patted my leg. "So, we need to start thinking about whether you want to do another round after this."

Wait? What? Hold on, Ms. Lippy. Another round? No one had ever said anything about another round. I thought today was supposed to be a better day. I had finally come to terms with six. I was feeling confident. Now you are telling me I have four and that I will probably have to go through another round?

I was officially in one of those dreams where you find yourself in a room with no doors. Where was Dr. Cheng? Did she know about what "Dr." Tammi was saying? This woman doesn't know me. Does she even know how to count?

I left in a hurry. Offended, upset, shocked. I needed to talk to Cheng, and I needed to talk to her now. I left a message for her and waited anxiously for her call back. I walked to my car and got in. I thought I was done crying. I thought I had passed the stage of bad news. After the last appointment, I had already used up all of the napkins in my car to blow my nose. I literally had to take off my sock and blow my nose in it. I wish I could say that was my low point. But I'm afraid we are just getting warmed up.

CHAPTER 9

MY CLIENT'S BALLS

Couples going through IVF have an unspoken understanding with each other. A code, per se. Like "I've been there" and "I'm here for you" and "We are going to be bonded for life." *Blah blah blah*. I get it. I love camaraderie in any form. But I don't think it gives you the Disney freakin' FastPass to skip the line and start talking about subjects you would never ordinarily talk about with strangers. It's like poking your head into someone's refrigerator without asking. You just don't go there.

I didn't know how comfortable I was going to be telling people that we were going through IVF. I was still trying to figure out how to tell myself half the time, let alone those around me. I was just not ready to be exposed yet. A few of our close family and friends knew, and I'm sure a lot of people were guessing. But I wasn't ready to advertise it. Maybe I was still in denial. Maybe I felt like I could squeak by without anyone really ever knowing. Maybe I didn't want people to look at me like I was damaged. Whatever the reason, I was just not ready to make an announcement to the world. Most days I was trying to just go on living my life. No one asked. It was my little secret, and to be honest, it felt right. Safe in the confines of my own body. Protected. Until that one day. The day I got the privacy ripped away from me. His name was Ted. And he had balls. And I was about to hear all about them.

Ted is a client of ours who comes by frequently to check on jobs he has in our plant. I don't see him often, but he pops into my office once in a while—an interaction that I never think twice about. We usually exchanged a quick hug. A pleasant hello. Maybe a "How's the family" and then we both rushed in our separate directions. I wouldn't think about the guy again until a few weeks later when the same interaction took place. But that day was different. When I saw him lingering outside my office, waiting for me to get off the phone, I had a feeling. You know the feeling. Like you can't avoid what is about to happen.

I hung up the phone, and just like I knew would happen, his head popped in the doorway. Ted was a very tall man in his early fifties. Rosy cheeks. Friendly face. He had this way of speaking where his lips would overly pronounce every word. Like he was on *Reading Rainbow* or something. He came in and said, "Vince told me you guys were having some...trouble."

I knew exactly what he was talking about, but my world started spinning. In a moment of defense topped off with panic I said, acting oblivious, "What do you mean?"

He looked around and then whispered, "The baby stuff."

There were so many things going through my mind. I was enraged that this information had leaked out. I was caught so off guard. I didn't want him to think that I was a damsel in distress who needed saving. I was fine. It was no big deal. For whatever reason, I didn't want to bond with him over this.

"We had trouble too, you know."

How was I supposed to react to that statement? Oh, really? That's great. Was it your fault or hers? I just said, "Oh. I didn't know."

Ted then came in and sat down. I leaned farther back into my chair, bracing for whatever was going to come next.

"I have to tell you the funniest story." He started to get even redder than normal, and I knew that the story was headed straight to "the jerkoff room." Much like the brain hides trauma from your consciousness, my attention started to wander in and out. I heard words like porn magazine and nurse and the cup. The misery kept getting worse. My insides were screaming, *No, no, oh God no. Don't go there, please don't.* My ears were burning, *Oh man, oh man, he went there.* The Doppler reading in my brain at this point was at a category 5 hurricane. Bring in the National Guard because I was never going to unhear any of what was just said. I didn't even know what his point was. *I jizz, too? Isn't IVF fun? Who doesn't like a good eighties porn?*

I just sat there. Responding in various tones of "oh" and "hmm" and "hmph." Waiting to be rescued. He finally finished up and walked out.

What the hell just happened? Did a client really come into my office and tell me a jerkoff story? Was that his idea of a motivational speech? Sure, I realized that he was just trying to connect—maybe make light of a sensitive issue. All I have to say is that if he ever comes to my home, I am locking the refrigerator door!

As the weeks went on, I would cringe every time I saw him. When he walked my way, my entire insides would tighten up as if someone was wringing me dry. Not even because of the balls story. Just because he "knew." I hated that he knew. I would rush through my interactions with him and avoid eye contact. I didn't want him to ask for an update. I didn't want to have to tell him it wasn't going well. And I definitely didn't want to hear "Ted's Balls: The Sequel." I hear it was a real nail biter.

CHAPTER 10

EGG HUNT

After forty-two shots, seven blood tests, four ultrasounds, three mental breakdowns, and two very bitchy weeks, I was ready for the retrieval. The key to the process is waiting to see how mature the smallest egg can get without losing the biggest. When the time is right, the doctor goes in and surgically removes all the eggs from the ovaries. Once the eggs are retrieved, they can try to fertilize them to create an embryo.

We were confirmed for 8 a.m. two days from now. Tonight, I was to receive what they call a trigger shot. The hormones I had been taking were preventing me from ovulating. Now I was going to take a medication that would force me to ovulate in forty-eight hours.

That night, we downloaded the instructions. I assumed the needle would be similar to the others. I could not have been more wrong. Jack read the steps and watched his lady friend on the videos again as I stared at the size of the trigger needle. It was huge. It looked like the kind of shot they show in Warner Bros cartoons. It was thick and large and scary as shit. Oh, and it was to be plunged right into the muscle in my butt. It had to pierce through the skin and through the fat to get inside the muscle.

I have two words for you, ladies: ICE PACK. A friend of mine who had gone through the procedure told me about this trick. *Shout out to Tara!* "Just put an ice pack on the injection site for ten minutes before you do the shot, and it numbs the pain." So that's what I did. For thirty minutes. "How long are you going to keep that thing on there for?" asked Jack.

"As long as it takes to never feel my ass again."

"A rhinoceros could lift you up by the butt with his tusk, and you wouldn't feel it."

"Well if you're so brave, why don't you jam it into your butt?"

"Do you think I want to stab you with this thing?"

"Well, you better enjoy it because it's the closest you're going to get to giving it to me in the butt."

"Very funny. And no, it's not."

"Yes, it is. Now stay focused, stabber jammer."

Jack put his game face on. He was in the zone. Barely talking. Reading and rereading his directions. You have to select the right area. It's the top outer portion of your butt muscle. He had to stab the needle in hard and fast and then pull it out a little to make sure not to draw any blood, which would mean that you hit a blood vessel. Such a mistake is rare, but they insist you do it that way. *(As if the shot alone wasn't frightening enough, they have to add that little ditty.)*

It was go time. He took the plastic slipcase off the needle and poked it into the vial of medication. "God, could they give you any less medicine in here?" he groaned as he struggled to get the needle to draw the amount of fluid needed. I could tell he was getting frustrated as his nerves were kicking in. Finally, he drew up one cc. He was careful not to cause any air bubbles. After the medication was safely drawn in the vial, he switched the needle. He secured it tightly. "Okay."

I leaned against the counter. I put all my weight on the opposite foot like Google told me to do. I closed my eyes and waited. My head was spinning. I was sweating. I had no idea what was in store here. I pictured that humongous thing piercing all those layers of my body one by one. Waiting for an update. "Dude, what's going on back there? You doing your taxes? What are you waiting for?!"

"Stay still," I heard him say patiently. "And...done."

"What? I had no idea it was even in there." I started crying and hugged him. I had been thinking about that particular shot for two weeks. "We did it. I'm not even sore! You did it, babe."

"No, you did it!"

"Wait, Jack, I'm not even sore. Are you sure you got the right spot?

Everyone said I would be sore. Is there a bruise? I don't see a bruise! Did you do it right?"

"I think I did it right. I mean, where else would I do it? How big is the butt muscle?"

"I think it's pretty big. Oh man, I have a fat butt. Do you think it reached the muscle because of my fat butt?"

We looked at each other in panic. These last two weeks of heartache would mean nothing if this shot didn't work. I spent the next nine hours, until I saw the doctor again, looking in the mirror at my butt—trying to feel where my muscle was. Clenching my butt back and forth one hundred times to make sure it worked. Nine hours later, when I could barely walk, it was clear he had stuck me good. We were on to the main show. The retrieval.

Early the next morning, I found myself watching the sun rise over the Hudson. I loved watching the steam come off the water on those brisk May mornings. Our apartment has a beautiful view of the river, and it always had a calming effect on me. Even today.

We arrived at the office early. We signed in and waited. It's always scary when you don't know what to expect. I looked out the window. That high up, the city looked so peaceful. As I sat there nervously, I thought of how many people were having a normal day.

When they finally called us, they took us to a room lined with a row of beds with curtains. They asked which bed I wanted because I was the first one. I chose one by the window. "That one. That one would be great."

I sat on the bed, and the first thing the nurse did was close the curtain that faced the window. As if to shut me out from the outside world—as if this whole process didn't do that enough on its own. I undressed, and they gave me a gown. I got into the bed and waited. In came nurse Tamika, with the personality of a diva rock star. I loved her immediately. She came in loud and strong. "Well, hello there, child. And how are we today?"

I was caught off guard by her enthusiasm but held onto it like a crutch. "I'm good. Little nervous but good."

"Oh, there ain't nothing to be worried about today, darling. I'm going to be right here with you. The sun is shining, and it's a good day to be alive." She was so right. It was a great day to be alive. It was all going to be okay. "Okay, my love, so this is what we are going to do. You are going to sit and relax. The anesthesiologist will be in soon to get you all IV'd up."

"Ugh, that's the part I've been worried about. Another needle. Does it hurt?"

I was expecting her to make me feel better, but she answered, "Oh, yeah girl, it hurts," she said as she kept on with her paperwork.

"I appreciate your honesty. So, when you say hurt, how bad do you actually mean?"

Before she could respond to me, she looked at Jack. "While this is going on, you, handsome sir, are going to go into that little room down the hall and do your umm-emmm-ummm into the cup."

She waved her hands from side to side as her body moved in this sexy wave-like motion. It was so politically incorrect. It was perfect.

I waved at Jack. "Go ahead, dear, go do your emmm-emmmm-emmm." Knowing she nailed it as she left us laughing, the diva dropped her microphone and exited the room. Not so happily, in walked the complete opposite human being, the anesthesiologist, who had about as much personality as a rubber glove: Dr. Patel.

She asked me a bunch of questions and then dug the IV into my arm with about as much tenderness as the Tasmanian devil. My girl was right, the initial stab hurt. But the pain soon passed.

While the nurses were getting ready for us, Jack sat with me and rubbed my head. I thought to myself how every day that you don't have to be doing something like this is a good day. Those mundane Mondays and Tuesdays that won't end, they're good because they are just normal days. They aren't one of the bad ones.

The nurse came in and said it was time. My eyes filled with tears, and I got that feeling in the back of my throat like I was about to cry. Not sure what prompted it. Saying goodbye to Jack felt really sad. I was all alone now. It was my time to perform.

They asked me to empty my bladder one last time and then walked me into the room. I was so happy to see Cheng. She was all suited up in her surgery gear. She had music going that was really quite pleasant. She asked me what I wanted to hear.

I said, "Really, the question is what do you want to be listening to!"

She put on something upbeat. I lay down on the table and waited. It's a weird feeling knowing that any second you are going to pass out. I felt light-headed just waiting, but nothing had entered into my system yet. I wondered if I would notice falling asleep. I wondered if it would hurt. I stared at the ceiling. And then...I woke up.

I was back in the bed I started in. The retrieval must be over. No one was around. I floated in and out of wooziness, but I was relieved that it was over. The nurse came in laughing. "Well, how is our little hugger?"

I had no idea what she was talking about but just answered, "Feeling pretty good."

The next face I saw was Cheng's. "Are you always that supportive?"

I looked around as the laughing continued around me. What the hell had happened in there? "Is there something I should know?" I asked with confusion.

Dr. Cheng answered "You came out of the surgery and started hugging all the nurses and telling them that it wasn't that bad and not to worry. We were hysterical. We couldn't get you to stop. You made it all the way down the hall before we could stop you."

"Oh man. Well, at least I wasn't naked."

"Well, you weren't completely naked..."

I just closed my eyes and put my hand to my head. At least everyone was having a good time. Unreal. I guess goofy is better than grumpy going on some Clomid-induced killing spree. It was comforting to know a happy person still lurked deep inside me.

When Jack came back in, Cheng updated us on what happened. "We were able to retrieve four eggs."

I immediately started doing the math in my head. What did this mean? We still had several stages left to go. They would perform the ICSI (intracytoplasmic sperm injection), which is the fertilization procedure where they take one sperm and insert it into the egg. We then had to wait six days for the eggs to mature. After that they would freeze the eggs and then send a small cell from the embryo for genetic testing.

Each stage tends to lose a few eggs along the way, and I only had four to begin with. There weren't many to waste. In my mind, I wanted three kids. I needed at least three good eggs. The nurse came in and gave me apple juice and crackers. It was time to go home. They would let me know tomorrow how many of the eggs successfully fertilized.

I had a good feeling, though. I had to root for these little guys, and I had all the confidence in the world that they would be strong. There was no reason for them not to be. When we got home, I fell asleep. Relaxed and calm. It was over.

The next day, Saturday, we waited for the results. It was torture. I firmly believed that we were going to nail this, but the time dragged on forever. I kept telling myself the hard part was over, and all we had to do was move forward and think positively.

We woke up early and drove out to Jersey to see my parents. Anything to distract us. I must have checked my phone every few seconds. We sat down to lunch. Vince and Grace came by. Everyone knew what was going on and did a good job of not bringing attention to it.

Grace was just starting to show a little baby bump. The irony was always tough to swallow, but I had to rise above that. She was very kind in those moments. I could tell she was uncomfortable talking about her pregnancy. I always felt bad about that. But I did appreciate the sensitivity.

After lunch, we were all talking around the table when I saw my phone buzz. NYCM appeared on the screen. I picked it up and ran outside. I heard Cheng's voice on the other end. She asked how I was feeling, but all I wanted was the result. Cheng said that of the four eggs, three successfully fertilized. I took a deep breath and thanked her. She said she would update us again in a few days to see how many were maturing.

I looked through the window and found the entire family staring at me, including Jack. I kept the phone to my ear as if I were still talking even though Cheng had already hung up. I could tell they were all waiting for my reaction, and I didn't know how I felt. Three was good. Four would've been better, but three was good, right? Why didn't it feel good? Was it selfish to have wanted all four?

I stood there for a few seconds longer, needing the time to figure out how to feel. I gave everyone the thumbs up and walked inside. I let them know the news.

Jack stood up and hugged me hard. I sensed that he was worried about me. My father, the eternal optimist, announced, "They are all going to make it. No doubt."

Grace agreed and said, "This is it, Brett."

But the looks from my mother and brother told a different story. Their faces showed what I was feeling. The truth was no one could wish this to happen. It wasn't like we could try harder and make this work. The end result was out of our hands. I never felt like I had less control in all of my life.

We had yet another hurdle to overcome: the maturing stage. They let the fertilized eggs mature for six days. What this means is that they want the egg cells to keep dividing until they can be frozen. The longer the egg keeps dividing, the stronger the egg and better it is for the transfer, which is the process of putting the egg, now fertilized, into the uterus. Cheng was going to give me an update in three days to see how it was going. My life was on pause.

There was something about this whole process that made me feel so run-of-the-mill—like everything I had done in my life to set myself apart as an individual didn't matter now. I felt like a big lump of science. It was an odd feeling. It was both comforting and scary at the same time. I realized that I couldn't do a thing to change the outcome. I could not work harder at some facet of this process to make it different. I could not face the fact that I was an IVF patient. A real one. As that name sank in, it became more and more devastating. I just couldn't fathom a world in which I was a girl unable to get pregnant. It didn't make sense. It made less and less sense as we got in deeper and deeper and received more and more bad news.

I was left feeling like I was living in someone else's reality. I didn't know where to turn. Everyone around me believed, as I once did, that I would be fine. Because, well, I have always been fine. I have always risen above. But how could they know now? They knew less than I did. The reality is getting pregnant was not something that positive thinking could change. The result was very black or white, and that is not how my brain is wired to think. I live in a world where I feel like I can will anything to happen. Feeling helpless was foreign to me. I didn't know how I fit into this whole process. I was simply another desperate patient in the waiting room, and everything was out of my hands.

Cheng called us two days later and reported that only two of the embryos were still dividing. We were down to two. Odds were not playing in our favor. With each lost embryo, my heart broke a little more. I had to stay positive for the other little guys, but it got harder and harder each time. Her news also meant that inevitably I was going to have to do another round of IVF. Another round of everything we went through, again. Even thinking about it was exhausting.

Two days later, we got the all-important call. I could tell that Jack heard me pick up the phone in the other room when the volume was muted on the TV. When the call was over, I hung up the phone and walked into the living room, where he was waiting anxiously. "We're down to one embryo." I started to cry. The loss of one more was devastating. "Only one little guy made it, Jack."

"I'm so sorry. Come here." He grabbed my head and pulled me toward his chest. "We still have one in the game, Brett. It's not over yet."

He continued to console me. "I believe in him. I know he can do this. Hold on, little guy." He stroked my head. "I feel like I know him already."

"Me too. Herbie." I said.

"Herbie?"

"Yeah, Herbie. The little embryo that could."

He sounded doubtful about this new idea. "That name doesn't sound like much of a fighter."

"Oh, don't let his name fool you. He's really understated like that."

"Oh, okay," Jack said, playing along. "Well, Herbie it is. Our little fighter."

I laughed though I could feel my heart still breaking inside of me. I nestled back into his chest. We felt like a family already. I never channeled so much energy into one little thing in all my life.

The next step was, they were going to do was freeze the embryo, take a cell off it, and send it for genetic testing for chromosomal abnormalities that would cause the embryo to miscarry. The sperm and the egg are supposed to both have twenty-three sets of chromosomes. Those chromosomes need to be equal. If they aren't, the embryo/baby could have defects that would cause it to not sustain a pregnancy to its full term. Depending on which chromosomes are deficient affects the severity of the defect.

Getting the results back would take seven to ten days, and waiting for these results was the hardest part yet. Jack and I believed in our little Herbie, though, and we would talk about him often in order to help the time go faster. "Do you think he's cold in the freezer?" I asked Jack.

"I think he's perfectly fine."

"Maybe we should go visit him. We could bring him little embryo gloves."

Jack laughed as he always did at my ten-year-old humor. Though we joked, we rooted him on with everything we had. We talked to him every night and imagined all the places he went during his journey to Boston to get tested. Herbie was a legend. A world traveler already. He wasn't going to let us down.

Whether we were in for another round of IVF or not, it felt good to know that we still had one in the game. I knew in my heart that this one would be healthy. It had survived all the other obstacles: the retrieval, fertilization, maturing. Herbie, our little embryo that could. He would shock the world. They say that at my age about half the embryos that go in for genetic testing end up being good. We had a 50/50 chance at this point, and we felt confident. Herbie had this in the bag. "A little embryo bag with little embryo toiletries."

"Okay, Brett, I get it."

↗ CHAPTER 11 ↖

INTERMIX

There's something about walking down a New York City street in those first few beautiful days of spring that can make you forget if you let it. One Saturday morning, I put the blinders on to the women with the strollers and the oversized diaper bags and allowed myself to get lost in my city. There's an odd beauty in realizing what a small piece of the world you are. Somehow in humbling myself, it made me feel alive. I could detach myself from all the emotions of trying to get pregnant. Walking so far that the stores started to blur together as I left the neighborhoods I knew farther and farther behind me. I could see peace in the chaos as I walked from block to block, admiring the different personalities of each new neighborhood. I found comfort in remembering that these streets replay the routines of the thousands of people who inhabit them every day as I'm replaying mine, making me feel less alone.

I jumped on the subway to make my way back downtown. (Ok, I actually took a taxi, but didn't me saying I took a subway make me sound so much more like a New Yorker? Let me have this moment.) So, I jumped on the subway to make my way back downtown. But before I could head home, I had to make one last stop—at a place where the sizes ran small and the people judged you from head to toe, a place that made me feel like a somebody while making me feel like a nobody. My favorite place in the city: INTERMIX. For those of you who don't know it, INTERMIX is a clothing boutique. They sell all the latest trendy clothes, and women all over New York City can be seen draped in them at any given West Village brunch spot. It's almost like a rite of passage. Though I was bloated and thought nothing would fit, I found myself wandering in.

When a sales rep approached me, she looked down at my stomach that was completely bloated from the hormones, and then back up and asked, "Are you expecting?"

"Yes. As a matter of fact, I am." I answered.

I don't know why I lied. Maybe I didn't want to get into the whole saga. Maybe it felt good to live in someone else's life for a moment. Maybe I just simply didn't want her to think I was fat. She then proceeded to say that she had the greatest dress for maternity. Caught in my lie, I tried to ignore her and show her that I wasn't interested, but she ran in the back so enthusiastically that I didn't have the heart to stop her.

When the rep returned, she was carrying a black dress on a hanger. It looked like a size zero fit for a thirteen-year-old. I had to laugh: there was no way that was going to fit me. But before I knew it, she was pushing me into a dressing room. I removed my clothes and saw my pale flabby body that hadn't been tended to in months—a bush that looked more like a jungle than a bikini line and pasty ashy skin that needed to be soaked in moisturizer and basked in the sun. I put my head through the dress and pulled it down over my body, careful not to paint it with my caked-on deodorant. The material was light, and it surprisingly formed around me.

The little bitch was right. It looked amazing. Well, it would've looked amazing if my stomach protruding out of it was actually a baby belly and not just bloating. I stared at myself in the mirror. I couldn't take my eyes off the reflection. I pushed out my stomach a little farther to see what I would look like pregnant. It was wonderful. I saw the vision. I saw the big picture. It felt like a sign—like this was going to work for me and Herbie the embryo was going to come through for us. The sight made me feel something deep inside. Excitement. Hope. Confidence.

I took the dress off and gave it back to the salesgirl. I thanked her and walked out. She'd never know how much more she had done for me than just handing me that dress.

I walked for a few blocks, thinking of all the amazing things to come. Those New York streets did for me exactly what I needed them to do. I reached the corner of Christopher Street and Seventh Avenue, where the subway station was. I walked right past the entrance, got into my yellow "subway," and headed home.

⚗ CHAPTER 12 ⚗

WHAT'S IN A NAME?

On Monday morning, I was at work. The hustle of the workday was a welcome distraction. Only five days had passed since our embryo had gone for testing, so when I got a call from a random number with Cheng's voice on the other end, I was caught off guard. She paused on the phone and then said, "The embryo didn't pass genetic testing. I'm so sorry."

She said it all so fast. Wait? Herbie? Our little Herbie? And just like that he was out of our lives forever. I was crushed. I hung up the phone and didn't know what to do. I never even conceived the possibility that he wouldn't make it. I mean, he was a fighter. Herbie the fighter. What's in a name anyway? I paged Vince, who was in the office next to me. He came in and shut the door.

I started crying. "He didn't make it."

The hurt that was filling my body was like nothing I had ever felt before. It was a combination of despair. And fear. And confusion.

And shock. It was pure sadness. Vince tried to console me. He sat by my side as I cried. There was nothing either of us could say. I called Jack and let him know what had happened. He stayed strong on the phone, but I knew he was hurting. Maybe I blocked out the idea that the embryo could fail. Maybe we humanized him too fast. No matter what it was, we were lost.

My immediate response was to go in and see Cheng and get right back in the game. I didn't want to wait. I needed to get this done, and there was no time to waste.

We went to see Cheng later that afternoon. As we sat in her office waiting for her to come in, we couldn't seem to break the silence that fell over us. Our confusion bounced off the walls over and over as we dwelled inside our own thoughts.

Cheng came in and sat down. "I'm so sorry. I really am." She laid a piece of paper down in front of us. "It would've been a boy."

Hearing that news killed me. Maybe it was picturing the baby as a boy. Maybe it was the fact that I always wanted a boy first. Either way, the news was awful.

"It had a chromosomal abnormality, and it would never have made it to term. It would've been severely mutated and would've miscarried. I am so sorry." Suddenly, a nurse paged Cheng, and she excused herself and walked out.

Jack and I sat there stunned, unable to speak to each other. I looked up at him. "It would've been a boy."

He looked back, somber. "Yeah."

"But that mutant ninja turtle thing, yikes. C'est la vie." As I waved it off, like who needs that? He looked up in shock that I had gone there. To our horror, we both started to laugh hysterically. All of our swirling emotions came out as laughter, but the release felt good. When Cheng came back in the room, she must have thought we were crazy. Maybe we were. But it felt good to laugh. All that mattered now was getting back in the game. Our hopes for Herbie might be over, but we were not giving up that easily.

Cheng walked us through what we could expect in the next round. She was going to keep the drug regimen the same. She wanted us to take a month for my body to heal. I wanted to get right back in the ring, but she cautioned us to wait. I had no choice but to follow her advice.

We got back to the apartment mentally exhausted. When we walked in the door, we discovered a package waiting for us. We brought it upstairs. We casually opened it to find a pineapple from Hawaii from a friend of ours, Sarah. She had gone through the IVF process as well and knew we were struggling. Pineapple is a fertility fruit and is supposed to help. During moments like these you have to count on the positive energy from your friends. It was the perfect gift. We had to reach within ourselves for more hope. We had to keep fighting. We were IVF patients. And there was only one way out because I was not ready to give up.

CHAPTER 13

OH, *THOSE* HORMONES

Cheng suggested we take a month off in between rounds; I was opposed, but I had no choice but to follow the doctor's orders. I didn't want anything to hinder our chances of being successful. The weather was right on the brink of where spring turns to summer. There was hope in the air. I felt more prepared for this round. I knew what to expect. I knew that we would have more success. I just knew it in my gut. My body was used to the grind now. Maybe we needed a round to get the routine down. The last one had been like a trial run. Cheng said we could try naturally if we wanted. Jack and I both heard her say it, but we never really discussed it. The idea of actually having sex and getting pregnant felt foreign to us. Maybe it would be the time that everyone talks about, when they didn't even try, had sex, and then surprise, it worked! After a few failed attempts though, it became clear that this would not be our reality. The winds of change became dead air as we sailed on to Round Two.

We soon were receiving drugs at the door again, and Round Two had officially begun. I had a hard stop to drinking, exercising, sex, caffeine, hot tubs, and pretty much anything else that made me a normal functioning person in society. It didn't matter. It was go time. I was in the state championships, and I was ready to play.

This time around, I started to feel the effects of the hormones much more than I had before. I was very bloated, for one. I hadn't had a bowel movement in almost a week and a half. My face looked tired and pale, and my chin started at my neck. Nothing was worse than the hot flashes, though. I would wake up in the middle of night in a pool of sweat and that was only when I was lucky enough to be in my own apartment. One night we went out with friends at a restaurant in SoHo, and I found myself stripping down at the table layer by layer. I repeatedly asked, "Is it hot in here? Are you sure it's not hot in here? No one feels that huh?"

I actually went in the bathroom just to pull my jeans all the way down to my ankles to get relief for a minute. I'm pretty sure I even moaned when they reached the bathroom floor. A SoHo bathroom is no place for a fragile female. No one cares what is going on with you. They'll kill you with their five-foot-ten-inch-tall waif death stare if you take one second too long in the stall. It's a dark, lonely place if you're bloated. Especially if you're in flats. Especially if you're taking too long in the bathroom. It's SoHo suicide.

Besides the physical discomfort, the emotional effects started to hit me hard. My moods soared up and down, and I didn't have any control over what I was feeling. My mother made up names for the moods. "Dolores" was really sad. On one of those days, I'd wake up and just not stop crying. My emotions got the best of me. The smallest setback could launch me into a puddle of self-pity.

"Matilda" was the opposite. She was a raging bitch. She'll find ya, and she'll kill ya. Matilda was definitely worse because I didn't know what she was capable of saying or doing. I would find myself barking orders at people at work or overreacting to the smallest problems. You wouldn't think mood swings are that big of a deal, but when you're running a company where its success is based on your demeanor, you better believe it becomes an issue. I found myself even sassing back to clients. It was a bad scene.

My brother started calling them Progesterone Bombs. He would hear me from his office launching one on someone and run in to stop me, but most of the time, it was too late. It got so bad that I realized I had to start telling a few people at work. The emotional swings occurred too often and, quite simply, were not me. On some days, I probably shouldn't have even been out in public.

On the day of my first follicle check, I was pretty much a beast, limping in with clothes I had torn through like the Hulk, breathing hard and grunting. I came in and sat on the table. Jack came with me this time. We were no dummies. There was no such thing as a casual appointment anymore.

When Dr. Cheng came in, I was nervous. I couldn't pretend to be strong. I knew this was our chance to redeem ourselves, and the thought of failure was scary. I sat up on the table. Cheng started with her magic wand. With each passing jerk inside me, I waited to see a little circle in the screen. I was stunned when she counted ONLY four. I couldn't believe that the numbers were not only low again but even lower than last time. That possibility never crossed my mind. My head started to spin again as disappointment welled up in my body. Combined with the hormones, I had no shot in hell of an acceptable, controlled reaction. I was a mess again.

Four follicles. As prepared as you think you are, nothing prepares you for bad news turning worse. Every time I went into that office, I should've anticipated news one-degree worse than what I was expecting. You never leave inspired; I will tell you that right now. Do not look to them to make you feel better. *I'm serious here.* This is a real warning. If I could make that statement run along the bottom of the page like a blizzard warning, I would. They are all rough appointments. And they are disappointing because you cannot predict what is about to come next. In my case, the issue was the number of eggs; other women were told about surprise surgeries they didn't see coming, or they learned their bodies didn't respond at all to the fertility drugs. They are little devastating detours that keep you off the direct path of what you really want. Buyer beware!

The fallout of this one hit way harder than I was expecting. I couldn't believe I was in this boat again, let alone being there in the first place. I was still in denial about even having to do this at all. Whose life am I living? How can I be this much more screwed up than every other girl I know? I mean, I don't even have allergies! Not only am I in IVF, but even the IVF isn't working. Who does that happen to! The frightening prospect of what was to come poured over me.

When I went back three days later for another check, they found only three follicles. The nurse asked if I wanted to bother going through with this round. As disappointed as I was with the count, I became protective and defensive. Matilda looked at her, as if to grab her by the throat and say, "Oh, we are going in there, bitch, if it's the last thing we do."

CHAPTER 14

YOUR NEIGHBOR'S FRIEND'S DOG WALKER

One thing I am learning very quickly is that some of the things in life that used to bring me such happiness and joy have become a source of complete and utter stress. I used to enjoy seeing family and friends, especially the ones I hadn't seen in a while. But now I dreaded going to parties and places where people could ask me questions that I was ashamed to answer. Worse than that, though is "the advice." The advice you get from all the geniuses who pretend to be an expert on everything you are going through. The funny part was, the people with the most kids thought they were the most helpful. Please, stop saying that you had "trouble getting pregnant with your third child" or that you "miscarried in between kids three and four." It's not the same, and it's a dagger in the heart when you try to sell it like it is. I had to suffer through child-bearing advice from a GOMO who had the luxury of planning when she was going to have her next baby. *After vacation? After Brian's wedding in Mexico? I always wanted a summer baby, so maybe I will wait until the fall.* They just didn't get it. It's the emptiness that hurts. The thought that you may never be able to look down at a baby who is your own. That's the hard part.

I've heard it all. "Well, if you stop stressing, it will happen." As if I was different than any other woman on earth who was ever worried about having a child. "My friend's neighbor's dog walker was trying for five years. Then they decided to adopt. Three days later, she was pregnant." What am I supposed to do with that story? What's the moral of that one? Stop at the orphanage on my way home from work so I can get pregnant? I mean, seriously? Thousands of other people have adopted without getting that result. It's not exactly an active fertility treatment they're researching in some underground lab in Siberia somewhere.

It was tough for me to hear advice from people who I'd witnessed crumbling over far less. As if they would be handling the situation any better than me, somehow insinuating that the feelings I was having were not justified. They'd tell me how to handle this: "Just stay positive, and it will all work out." How do they know it will work out? Were they in the doctor's office with me when I was told that my IVF procedure didn't work? Did they see the results of my tests? It drove me insane and left me acting very defensively.

"Why don't you just use a surrogate?" "Why don't you just use an egg donor?" That one hurt the most. As if there is absolutely no mental process to get through to accept the fact that you can't have your own natural child before exploring that option. This one was rough, and it broke me every time. It's not that I think people were being insensitive, I just don't think they really realized how frightening and heartbreaking every other option felt other than having your own child. I also don't think they realized how insulting it was to assume that the emotional consequences of those options were so easy to come by. It felt like their response was too casual for such a weighty issue. Maybe I would, maybe I will. But it still wore on me. At first, I could play it off and just yes people, but the deeper I got into it, the more it bothered me. Maybe there was something inside of me that knew they were right. Maybe the thought of that was terrifying. Maybe I was still in denial. Or maybe it was just none of their fucking business.

⌁ CHAPTER 15 ⌁

THE GRILL

The annual high school barbeque. This is a day once a year when all of my old friends and their husbands and children meet up and have a cookout at someone's house. What started as a drunk fest for singles years ago became a party with married couples and the occasional newborn. Now it has escalated to essentially a children's Chuck E. Cheese's party with a few exhausted adults standing around. I was on the fence about going from the start. Each day closer brought more and more anxiety. I didn't want to have to answer the questions as to why we didn't have children yet. I didn't want to see everyone and their perfect families. I didn't want to hear them complain about their trivial kid problems that I would do anything on earth to have. It hurts to see your dream lived out by everyone else—to feel like the only woman who couldn't give her husband what all these other women could.

Besides that, I felt bloated, pale, and drained. I couldn't even drink because I was in cycle. In fact, I would have to bring my injections to the party and do them there. It was a rough week with all our bad news, and I didn't know if I had the energy. Deep down, I was just embarrassed. Embarrassed to be me. Disgusted to be labeled as the girl who wasn't quite so great after all.

The party was being held at one of my best friend's houses. I had opened up to Erica about everything that had been going on. She and I discussed my reluctance to go, and after talking with her at length, we decided that the party would be good for me. I would be surrounded by friends who loved me. Besides, if I stopped being who I was, then where would that leave me? Further inside a life that I didn't recognize? I mustered up the courage and the energy and decided to brave it.

That morning, I put together an outfit that tried to scream, "I'm still cool because I don't have kids." I went with the "I didn't try" look, even though it took me about an hour and thirty-five outfit changes to achieve it. Though I hate being the girl in heels at a BBQ, I had no choice. When your thighs start to mesh in with your knees, it's definitely time for a little height.

It was a beautiful day, a little cool, but sunny. Cars were lined up and down the block when we pulled in. I could hear the music and voices in the backyard. I took a deep breath and got out of the car. Jack grabbed my hand, and we forged ahead. We had to gingerly walk down a hilly slope on the side of the house. This was sure to be an interesting entrance in platform heels.

I turned the corner and saw all the familiar faces of my friends. One by one I was greeted with a big hug. I made my way through the crowd. I couldn't help but notice the kids running around everywhere, but I felt good. I could do this.

I made my way through the crowd with my handsome husband by my side. Each passing conversation brought up laughs about the old days and jokes about how hectic everyone's lives are. Not one person pressed me about my situation. They asked about work, the new house, and my family. But they didn't touch the missing kid thing. They hugged me longer than usual, and I saw the compassion in their eyes. They cared too much to ask. They didn't selfishly pry. I grabbed on to that like a lifeboat in the middle of the dark ocean. It was breath in my lungs, and it felt refreshing. But most of all, it felt freeing.

An hour into the party, Vince and Grace showed up. Grace was beautiful pregnant. Bright-eyed, slender, with a little baby bump. As soon as they walked in, everyone was eager to talk to her and Vince about the baby. They were owed that attention. But it was hard. I'm not going to pretend that it wasn't. I kept maneuvering my way around the backyard, trying to steer clear of any comment that would send me into a hormonal spiral. I found Jack in the crowd. It was almost 5 p.m. at this point and probably a good time to break away and do my injection. I grabbed my purse, and we headed to the upstairs bedrooms.

We had to do two injections this time, and I cringed inside, hearing the noises of the children outside as Jack was getting ready to stab me in the stomach. It was those moments where it felt the most unfair. I had to try to stay strong.

When he finished the second injection, I noticed a little blood seeping through the skin. I folded some toilet paper over it and hoped that it would do the trick. I wrapped the needle up and shoved it in my bag to dispose of later. He looked at me and kissed me. "Are you okay?"

"I think so. Yeah. I'm okay. I mean I'm good. I mean okay. But good."

He smiled at me and rubbed the back of my head like he always does when he's getting a kick out of some little thing I am doing.

I made my way back down to the party. Taking deep, long breaths and trying to bounce back into the swing of things. And then it happened. She happened. Camila.

Camila is a California gal who married my friend Tom. She claimed she was a movie producer when really all she did was locate props for a studio. She was one of those people who got off on prying the uncomfortable out of you. She kept trying to catch my eye, and from the beginning, I knew she wanted a piece of me, but I was able to avoid her for the most part. She must have known what was going on with us, and she had that look like she wanted to talk about it. She prided herself on being a psychology major and would always try to go all therapist on me.

I finally ended up cornered by the food table, and I had nowhere left to hide. She launched right in. After making one comment about the weather, she immediately jumped in with this story about how she was going through IVF, too. *Camila?* I couldn't believe it. I looked at her in astonishment. Could she be dealing with what we were dealing with? In that brief moment I felt such a sense of alliance with her. Like maybe she did know what I was going through. And then...she kept talking. What I came to realize fast was that she was not going through IVF, she was freezing her eggs. She went on and on about how she didn't think it was so bad and how she didn't really know what the big deal was—that it was lucky even to be able to plan when you would get pregnant. I couldn't speak. I was at a loss for words.

Uncomfortable with where the conversation was headed, I tried to move away, but she kept at it. She went on about how she barely felt any effects and how she had frozen fifteen eggs and she could now wait and not have to feel rushed to have kids. You know because of her work schedule and blah blah blah. I kept thinking how unfair it was that she got to choose and how insensitive it was that she did not recognize the difference. I didn't know what to say. All I could think about was how badly I wanted the conversation to end.

"How did it go for you?" *How did it go for me?* Did she mean, how is it still going for me? I couldn't believe that she was actually comparing my situation to hers. The tears, the ups, the downs. If retrieving the eggs was all I had to do, I would do it daily. But what about the testing? What about the disappointments? What about the lack of choice? What about the lying in bed never knowing if you are ever going to be able to have your own child? And then you have this girl going on and on as if she had just gotten a freaking bikini wax. It felt horrible inside. I didn't know what to do.

She kept intruding and, without a choice, my emotions took over. "Well, it's actually been the worst year of my life, but I don't really feel like talking about it."

Then I sprinted off. I didn't even know where I was sprinting to. I saw Erica in the distance. I knew I'd be safe there. My best friend. My confidant. One of my people. I dashed to her and tried to tell her what happened. She looked at me and stared. She wasn't getting it. "Don't you think you're being a little oversensitive?" she finally murmured.

I couldn't believe what I was hearing. I was unable to speak. I walked away and tried to find the first bathroom I could. My head was spinning. My tears were brimming in my eyes, and I knew I was in a race against gravity. I ran up the stairs and started opening doors, trying to find a bathroom. I found one by the kids' rooms, closed the door behind me, draped myself over the sink, and started to cry.

When I could finally lift my head up, I looked at myself in the mirror. I was unrecognizable to myself. As I looked down in the sink, I saw toothbrushes in the shape of Disney princesses and towels with little hoods on them. All of the strength I had mustered to walk into that party was gone in one fell swoop. I wasn't even safe with my friends.

I realized that even friends were not able to understand, and it wasn't necessarily their fault. I felt more isolated than ever before. I found myself hoping that someday Camila would understand how she made me feel.

I heard a little tap on the door. I panicked. "I'll be right out." And then I heard, "It's me. Grace." Just with the way she said it, I knew she knew what had happened. I opened the door. She came in, shut the door behind her, pulled me in, and didn't let go. I cried like a baby in her arms. I told her my story. She held my hands as I went on and on. My blubbering may have sounded like gibberish to her, but she listened and held me and confirmed that what I was feeling was right, regardless of anything else. I wasn't as alone as I thought.

I heard the girls calling out my name from the front lawn. I washed my face, Grace dabbed a little blush on my cheeks, and I ran down to meet them. They were all lined up with their kids in front of an ice cream truck. They were waiting for me to take the group picture. I jumped in on the end. I looked down to make sure I wasn't stepping on a toddler and saw that the blood from my injection had seeped through my silk shirt. I quickly hid it with my hand. By the seventeenth attempt, the picture was finally snapped.

Not knowing where to go next, I looked up and saw Grace in the distance with my bag and hers. She looked at me and smiled. She started saying her goodbyes, making up a story about a family affair we all had to attend later that night. Vince and Jack weren't far behind. It was the sweetest sight I could've possibly seen. I'm not sure I ever really thanked her for that moment. Maybe I just did.

CHAPTER 16

THE SUN WILL COME OUT TOMORROW

My mother came with us to retrieval number two. With four mature follicles growing, it was sure to be a good day. We were hopeful. Jack had to get back to work after the procedure, and my mom was going to spend the afternoon with me as the anesthesia wore off. The number of blood tests and doctors' appointments throughout this process is intense. The late-to-work mornings and the random days off because of procedures were tough to manage. It's an odd side effect you don't think about. Jack and I are both people who don't take random days off from work for no reason. We are committed to our jobs, and it has always been a priority for both of us. We had to manage our workloads around this entire private whirlwind going on. We tried to spare afternoons and hours when we could by getting the earliest appointments in the day when available and trying to limit the amount of days off when we could swing it. My mother came in for the tag team this time.

My mother is a cool, tall blonde who looks about twenty years younger than she is. She is brave and tough but very warm and motherly as well. She had handled all of this so far with such grace and style—always there to field a host of crazy calls, tears, and hormones. She was more than willing to jump in the car and meet me anywhere I needed her to be. I was happy to have her at my side.

The procedure was scheduled for 9 a.m. I had told my mom to show up around ten but, like I knew she would be, she was already sitting there, ready, when we walked in. She stood up right away and bounced toward us. "There she is!"

"Mom, how long have you been here? You look pretty settled in."

"You know, I got here at seven just to be safe. You never know with city traffic." The thought of "city traffic" was one of my parents' top fears in life. Though it was unnecessarily early, and though Jack had a look of panic on his face knowing that he was about to ejaculate into a cup with his mother-in-law twenty feet away, catching a glimpse of her face before heading in meant all the world to me. She had with her a collection of crossword puzzles, magazines, and snacks—as if she was ready for the retrieval, transfer, *and* the birth. She was so sweet. Just knowing she was there made me feel better.

I gave her a hug. "Okay, well, we're going to go look for your future grandchild. Wish us luck!" I exclaimed, trying to lighten the mood. I didn't want her to sit out there and worry about me.

"You don't need luck. You've got this." She smiled at me and gave me a big fist pump in the air.

The vibe was positive, and she was happy to be there for us. I wanted her to look back on this day and remember me as brave, but the truth was, I was petrified. Maybe I was trying to put her at ease. Enduring my rattled nerves was hard enough, and I was uncomfortable putting that stress on other people—even Jack. But I guess certain people are stuck right in the middle of it with you, and Mom sure fits in that category. I gave her a quick hug, careful not to linger too long as I fought the urge to tear up. "See you in a few hours."

"See you in a few hours. Hang in there."

Two hours later, we were done. I saw my mom's face through the crack of the open door as we walked out. She jumped up quickly, excited to congratulate us and anxious to hear how it went. Even from across the room, I could tell she could read the pain on my face. "They only retrieved two eggs."

Her smile subsided. I could tell she didn't know how to react. "Okay. That's good. It only takes one."

I appreciated her trying to be positive, but I could see in her face that her heart was breaking for us. It's much different to experience the news on the front lines than to hear about it over the phone. It's harder to show positivity when you're staring at negativity. It's hard to know what to do and how to react when you don't have the time to soak in what it all means. I've noticed when I talk to people about it, they want to lift you into a positive place as soon as they can, especially when that's what they are used to seeing from you. Maybe the undercurrent of deep sorrow is too uncomfortable for them. Maybe it's too uncomfortable for me.

In any case, it's not easy to truly understand. It's much easier to hang up the phone and keep living your life.

Seeing the glow drain out of my mother's eyes was hard for me. I knew she was struggling to comfort me while also trying to lighten the mood. But this wasn't our first rodeo, and the truth was getting harder to hear.

I was emotionless. I felt empty. I couldn't speak. I just wanted to go home.

Mom quietly gathered her things and walked behind us as we made our way out. Jack draped his arm over my shoulder as we shuffled toward the elevator. When we got downstairs, he hailed us a taxi. I knew he was worried about me. I just couldn't find the words to reassure him today. "Tell me something so I know you're okay," he said as he helped us into the cab.

"I'm okay. I really am. I just want to go home."

I didn't want him to have to go to work with this massive weight on his shoulders. He had a speech to give in front of hundreds of people. I didn't want him to worry about me. He kissed me as he shut the door. I could tell he didn't want to leave me.

As we started to drive away, I turned to the window and just gazed out stiffly. After an uncomfortable six minutes of silence, I turned to my mother. "There were only two eggs. I just can't believe there were only two." She looked at me and waved me in toward her. I dropped my head on her lap and started to cry. She ran her hands through my hair.

"You're still in it."

"Where do we go from here? With only two, the odds are so far from being in our favor."

"One step at a time, Brett. One step at a time."

When we got to the apartment, my mother made me a bed on the couch like she used to do when I was home sick from school as a little girl. There was something so calming about having her take care of me.

I fell asleep, and when I woke up, she had lunch set up at the table. "Thank you for being here, Mom. You have no idea how much it means to me."

"You know, Brett, there is so much more to be being a mother than just getting pregnant. I know this feels like everything right now, but I promise you this, you will look into the eyes of your child someday, no matter how you got there, and know that it was worth all of this."

"I can't believe there are only two eggs. It keeps hitting me."

"What will be will be."

I knew what she was saying, but I didn't stop analyzing and obsessing. These two eggs were already fighting daunting odds, but I couldn't lose hope. Hope is a funny thing. Without it, the hole you feel inside is too deep and too dark to fathom. With it, you run the risk of heartbreaking disappointment. It's a hard balance to strike. I was not ready to let go of my hope. I held on to it, trying hard to not let it slip out of my grasp. But it was getting slippery.

When we found out six days later that only one of the two embryos had survived through the week, I knew that hope was all I had left. We found ourselves in a waiting game once again for the genetic testing results to come back. At this point, I didn't know what to feel. I wanted to feel positive that we had a little player still in the game. But a part of me had to separate myself from wishing the embryo would turn into a baby because it was too painful when the results came back negative like last time. Regardless of what I wanted, I could not change the result of that genetic testing. It was either going to pass or not.

I didn't want people to think I was being negative, but I didn't have the luxury of thinking everything will work out perfectly.

> *I am starting to feel confused. My nature is to think positively, but it's not based on anything real. I know Jack doesn't want me to get my hopes up. I think it's starting to really weigh on him how sad I've been. I see his heart breaking for me and for himself. Sometimes I forget that he's going through this, too. Is that weird? It's like I don't have room for his sadness too. I have too much of my own. I don't even know how to begin to deal with his at the same time. I don't know how to console us both. I feel like we're both in the fetal position, waiting for the tornado to pass, and there's nothing we can do. You sit? You wait? You pray to a god that you have barely talked to before? You hope? You hope.*

A few days later, I found myself stunned at my desk once again after the results came in that the egg didn't pass the genetic testing. I stared blankly at the wall for what felt like hours. I didn't know how to identify with the blackness dwelling inside me. Two rounds officially over, and we had nothing.

Hearing a knock at my office door, I immediately scrambled to pretend I was busy. I picked up my phone with no one on the other end and held it against my ear. My receptionist peeked in and signaled that she had something for me. Before I could brush her away, from behind the door came a bouquet of flowers. I was so caught off guard. I couldn't imagine who these were from and why. She laid them on my desk and walked out. I just stared at them, afraid of what the card would say. Maybe I was mistaken for someone who had their shit together—for someone who was accomplishing things. Whoever they were from, I didn't deserve them.

I opened the card. "The sun will come out, tomorrow. So, you've got to hang on 'til tomorrow." – *Love Cousin Jaci.*

My cousin. My blood. The one who used to make up commercials with me in the bathroom when we were kids. She didn't know the details of our latest round, but she didn't need to. Seeing those words on that card touched something deep inside me. I realized that for the first time the people in my life did not just care for me; they had started to carry me. I had to keep going. They weren't giving up, so neither could I, even if I wanted to. Even though my eyes were burning. Even though my heart was shattered. Even though my body was exhausted and bruised. Even though fear radiated through me like nothing I had ever felt before. Even though I was officially someone else.

I took a rose out of the bunch and placed it on my computer. It was a symbol of all I had left, of who I once was. I had to fight for her. That's what she would want from me.

CHAPTER 17

A VERY, VERY, VERY FINE HOUSE

We bought a house. We actually bought it a few chapters ago, but I wasn't ready to tell you. We also bought a Volvo big enough for an army. Don't ask. Back to the house. We were driving around one day and saw it, fell in love with it, and bought it. That was basically how it went down. We both always had the vision of raising our family outside the city. We both grew up in houses with front lawns and big backyards where you could play sports on the weekends. We never discussed a timeline, but we had an unspoken understanding. At the time, we didn't think there would be an issue with having a baby. It had never crossed our minds for a second.

We were staying at my parents' house in New Jersey for New Year's weekend. We had a little time to kill and were driving around the area. We found a house online that was nearby, and we wanted to take a drive and see it. It was something we often did, just for fun. When we drove by this one, it had a "for sale by owner" sign outside. We called the number on the sign, never thinking someone would pick up.

A raspy older man's voice picked up on the other end. I couldn't believe it. When we asked if it was okay if we came by, he said come on in. I'll never forget pulling into the driveway for the first time. The house was beautiful and unique. It was a stone house that had different types of trees all around it. It looked like an old English manor. It was every girl's dream.

While Jack turned off the car and jumped out, I sat in the car for a few seconds. Frozen with an odd fear that this could become a reality. We headed along a perfectly manicured pathway to the house. With each pace closer to the front door, I felt farther and farther from New York City. I always knew we would leave, but I never really thought it would be so soon. I'd had this vision of having a newborn in the city, pushing a stroller along the river with my oversized coffee. But this house—this house seemed perfect.

We knocked on the front door. Maybe we would hate it. Maybe it would be so old and dark that we couldn't bear it. The man opened the door, the afternoon light shined in, and the rest is history.

The place had us at hello. It wasn't just a house. I saw us living there. The front door opened onto a big welcoming foyer with a grand staircase. It was easy to picture our children running down it with bare feet anxious to meet our guests. As we walked through the empty rooms, it had a very warm feel, even in the cold

December weather. To the right was a dining room that could easily accommodate my big Italian family every holiday. There were no curtains on the windows, but they reminded me of the house where I grew up. I remember hiding in the curtains when people came in to sit for Christmas dinner. Getting curtains was a must.

We wound our way toward the kitchen. The kitchen. Oh lord, the kitchen. It was big and bright. There were windows everywhere that faced the backyard. I could imagine baseballs being launched across the yard as I'd yell to everyone to come inside because dinner was ready.

We made our way upstairs. The first room must have been the owner's son's room. It was bright blue and had a little built-in desk in the corner. It was sweet. That's where all the homework battles would happen. The next room was yellow with sweet flowers painted on the ceiling. This was obviously a little girl's room. It had a bathroom connected to it. I always wanted my own bathroom growing up. My daughter was going to be one lucky gal, I'll tell you that much. The next room looked like it was two rooms in one. Possibly one for a play room and one for the beds. Maybe we would put the twins in there, and they could wreak havoc. It was all making sense. I saw the vision. It made me feel excited and rejuvenated.

The master bedroom was downstairs. Its placement stressed me out a little. I pictured our kids having a nightmare and then having to come all the way down the stairs to wake us up. Maybe we would sleep upstairs when they were young. I could picture them running into our bedroom one by one and jumping on our bed to wake us up.

The house just felt right. Our house. The house that our children would call home. Imagining the remnants of times past made me feel so lucky to be at the beginning of our story and not at the end.

When we got back in the car, we called my parents to tell them the news, knowing for sure they would be ecstatic to finally have us closer to them. The silence on the other end of the phone proved otherwise though, and I was left feeling like we were doing something dreadfully wrong.

The owner wanted a delayed closing. We were in no rush, so we figured April would be perfect. That timing would give us some time to get our affairs in order. We came up with a plan to do some work on the house and move in around July. And of course, by then, we would have a baby on the way, so the wait was going to make much more sense. I would be closer to work and my family. Jack would have a longer commute, but it made sense for me to be closer for the baby since my job could be more flexible and having family close by would be an obvious help. Life would no longer center on late nights at the bars and brunching along Washington Street. We would focus on our family and the next stage in our lives.

As the closing date came closer, though, I became more anxious. Jack and I never spoke about it, but our unspoken understanding to move to the suburbs suddenly became the elephant in the room. We knew it was the right move and one that we both wanted ultimately. But it forced us to confront the fact that we still weren't pregnant while we were moving into a house built for the goddamn Brady Bunch.

The closing took place on a gorgeous Friday afternoon—one of the first warm days of the year. The city would've been on fire with lines at all the outdoor rooftops, everyone sneaking out of work early, text streams starting at ten in the morning discussing where everyone was going to meet up, and girls in their newest spring outfits, though there was still a little chill in the air. That didn't matter. It was spring, and it was time to be social again— time to reintroduce yourself and your open-toed shoes back into the world.

We drove from the lawyer's office to the house with keys in hand. It was just the two of us. I was in leggings, bloated from our last round of IVF. We pulled in. Conversationless. Tanless. Emotion- less. And most of all, childless.

✦ CHAPTER 18 ✦

GREAT SCOTT

We moved. We moved? We MOVED. I don't know which inflection I want for this. I don't even know which inflection I am feeling. It has been a rough start to the summer. I've been crying like a baby since we left Warren Street, Jersey bound. I feel bloated. It's July, and I've been wearing the same three outfits since May. I've had my hair tied back in this tight bun since Memorial Day. I have the sex appeal of a chicken. The skin around my mouth is dry and raw. Not sure what that is. I just learned that it's more expensive to paint your garage floor than it is to genetically test a human embryo, and I haven't shit in six days. Have you ever had to answer "prunes" to your father-in-law's question of "I'm running to the store, does anyone want anything?" So yeah, that happened. All that, and of course, the two completely unsuccessful waste of time, money, and energy rounds of IVF that I suffered through. Blow all that out of your piehole, you skinny Lululemon New York mommy that I was supposed to be.

What came with moving to Jersey, other than bugs that are not roaches and stores with parking lots, was Dr. Scott and RMA

(Reproductive Medicine Associates of New Jersey). Cheng was out, and Dr. Scott was in. We decided to switch doctors because of the move. He also had the reputation of being the best. He had been recommended to me by so many people. Everyone said he was the guy to see. He had been written up in all kinds of articles and written a few books of his own. A change at this point would be good. Maybe he could help us in ways that Cheng and her yoga-pants-wearing team of characters weren't qualified to do.

When I told Cheng we were leaving her practice, she didn't seem all that disappointed. Maybe she knew I would screw up her success rate, and she was happy to see me go. Maybe she understood the circumstances. Maybe she said goodbye to me and kept living her life without a second thought. Whatever it was, I was dying to get to this appointment and to hear how Dr. Scott would diagnose our situation.

Jack and I walked into a huge complex, all of which belonged to RMA. There was a real live parking lot where only people associated with IVF walked in and out. It was refreshing. It was like a safehouse. We walked into a huge waiting room with about forty-five chairs of all shapes and sizes inside. Different versions of living room décor: some leather chairs, some couches. They felt like little individual huddle rooms to regroup in. Soon they called our name, and we walked into Dr. Scott's office. It was decorated all in wood with awards and framed magazine covers all over the walls. It felt like a museum of sorts. Dr. Scott walked in. He was of average size. Fair skinned. Warm face. Casual demeanor. He greeted us with a firm handshake and a nice smile, putting us at ease immediately. We started to tell him our tale in as much detail as we could. He had our file in front of him and kept verifying our story saying, "I see that here." "Yes."

After twenty minutes of updating him on our journey, he closed the file and pushed it to the far end of his desk. He took out a piece of blank paper and a pen. He started to explain to us in simple words but distinct detail about the process and what actually happens inside a female's cycle throughout her life. There were no generic PowerPoints, there was no bang out run through. It was him talking to us, human to human, about what happens to our bodies as time goes on. There was a decency in his tone and a sincerity in the way he paused in between sentences.

"Everyone's cycle is different. Your age can provide guidelines, but it does not dictate the progression of your cycle necessarily. Women begin to menstruate at different times, and they go through menopause at different times. It has less to do with age and more to do with where you are in your own personal cycle."

The way he was explaining it made me feel less like IVF was unfair and more like this was simply what I had to do. I was not part of some big test with other women my age where everyone else passed and I didn't. Getting pregnant this way would probably have always been my truth. He went on and on, taking as much time as we needed, making sure we understood.

I had all kinds of questions. "So, Doctor, I've heard that acupuncture helps. Does acupuncture help?" "There is this guy in Madison who specializes in fertility. I could go there." "Does diet play a role? I'm pretty healthy, but I do eat a lot of pasta. I heard gluten isn't great for fertility. Does gluten affect the results?" "I sometimes get stressed at work. Could stress play a role?"

He paused "Brett," he said as he leaned forward and touched the center of his desk as if he were touching my hand, "This is not your fault."

I stared at him, stuck inside his words, not fully willing to accept what he was saying. Not even knowing what feeling was released inside me as a response. "But in terms of increasing my chances, are there ways that—"

"Listen to me again: this is not your fault."

I looked into his eyes and started to cry. I suddenly knew what I was feeling. It was the guilt leaving my body. Relief from a burden I didn't even know I was carrying.

"I know this process is hard. There are three things at play here: the mother's health, the father's sperm, and the eggs. There is nothing you have ever done or can ever do that will change the quality of those eggs. So, stop blaming yourself. That was decided way before you were born."

For the first time, I felt understood. I felt like someone got it—as if he was validating in a few sentences everything that I had been feeling. It made me want to scream, "YES, YES, finally someone who gets it!!" I wanted to jump up and kiss him from across the desk. Instead I just kept crying.

"Do you have any other questions? Please ask anything at all."

I asked the only question left, the one that I desperately needed the answer to. "Do you think we have a chance? I mean, do other people come here after two failed rounds?"

"All I can say is that you wouldn't be here if there wasn't an issue. Everyone who comes here is here for a reason. So, let's get all the data we can. With only two rounds behind you it's hard to make any conclusions just yet. But I will tell you this: I will be honest with you. We have to trust each other."

Trust him? I wanted to marry him! I looked deeply into his eyes: "I promise."

We started with an ultrasound. In that short amount of time, he concluded that the opening of my uterus was slightly smaller than usual and that during my retrievals, I could be damaging good eggs. I appreciated the personal treatment, not feeling like part of an IVF factory. He was already studying my individual body and trying to make conclusions based on what he saw.

He went into detail about how the quality of the egg is determined long before a retrieval. There is nothing we can do to change the quality of an egg. Especially as we get older, fewer and fewer eggs are usable, and more are damaged. The real key is to get as many eggs safely out of the body in the hopes of not damaging a quality egg in the process. Another point that I was really into: he said that the quantity you pull is not as important as the quality. That made these meager egg hunts I had endured for the past few months feel more positive.

Dr. Scott walked us into a room where we waited to sign some paperwork. I looked over at Jack, who had a glow to his face. "Are you feeling what I'm feeling, Brett?"

"Like I'm in love with Dr. Scott?"

"Yup."

"This is it, Jack. This is it."

The door opened and in walked Nurse Adrienne. I could tell she had worked with Dr. Scott for years just by her confidence in the routine. She came in and buzzed through the legal work. She jumped from subject to subject, laying down the law with each new topic: drugs, insurance, waivers. When we were done, I felt like a tornado had just whirled through the room, and when it departed, I had a stack of thirty copies of paper with my signature on them next to me giving them consent to do God knows what.

She closed the folder and handed it to me. As I tried to take it, she didn't let it go. "Are we clear about everything?" As she raised her eye up in the air. She was very regimented, like a drill sergeant. This woman had her shit together, and I wasn't about to disappoint her.

"Yes, I think I'm good."

She let go of the folder, and I fell back a little as she left the room. I looked over at Jack. "Well, I see who wears the pants in this relationship." He laughed.

After we left, I felt a renewed faith in our efforts. We were ready to move forward with round three. I left there feeling more hopeful than ever before. I was finally in good hands, and I was starting to feel fresh life pumping back into my body. I couldn't wait to get started.

As we drove home, we got a call from Jack's brother and sister-in-law. I was surprised to hear from them. I picked up, and they started with some small talk. But somehow I knew what they were about to say: they told us they were pregnant. I was happy for them, but hearing their good news quickly rekindled my despair. It was an unwelcome reminder that our problem still loomed in front of us. I stayed strong and happy on the phone. For them. For Jack. For the strong, brave woman I was trying to be. I did appreciate that they told us privately, giving me the courtesy of soaking in the news on my own.

When we got home, Jack ran inside to take a work call. I stayed in the car. Still. Stunned. My grandmother said that sometimes when you're about to lose it, you need to go into the bathroom, shut the door, put a towel over your face, and have an ugly cry. And that's exactly what I did.

Then and there I decided I was not going to let this next round get the best of me. I even decided to do the shots on my own. It was empowering in a way to take matters into my own hands. It also gave me much more flexibility, especially with Jack's having to commute into the city. I made an entire syringe station on our beautiful new dining room table. Wipes, tissues, and Band-Aids on one side, various-sized needles on the other. The room had a huge window that we hadn't put curtains on yet, and I'm sure our new neighbors had quite a show. They would for certain think we were drug addicts.

I didn't care. It felt good to see the sunlight. I was feeling really good. I was trying my best to ignore the disappointments during all that had happened and tried to focus on moving forward. We were in the trusty hands of Dr. Scott, Nurse Adrienne, and their dream team. Maybe the new team was the start of a really magical change. A change we deserved.

CHAPTER 19

SUMMER DRUGGIN'

By the time round three was in full effect, so was summer. We decided to head to the shore for the weekend. The weather was supposed to be perfect. My parents' house at the beach, which was typically a madhouse where cousins from all over New Jersey came to crash, was surprisingly vacant. Those weekends were amazing, and I used to live for them. But I needed some peace. I needed some quiet time. Not dealing with anyone outside the immediate family would be a great escape, and this weekend had the makings of being exactly what I needed.

Along with the little vacation from reality, Jack and I would have some time to get back on track. We had been drifting apart lately, connecting where we could but retreating further and further into our private worlds of hurt. We would have these words of encouragement and hugs for each other. But I was no dummy, and neither was he. This was all taking a toll on us in ways that I don't even think we realized at the time. Dinners started to get quieter, and I found myself relieved when it was bedtime. Some days felt like I was just going through the motions. But that was okay for the time being. Emotionless was better than despair. Anything was better than the unspoken despair.

We packed all our injections carefully in a big cooler and headed south. Vince and Grace were going to come down too, as well as my parents. I was excited for the distraction and really looking forward to some good old-fashioned laughs within the nest. Being around people who knew what we were going through was such a relief.

I hated feeling like all eyes were on me, especially when the topic of having a baby was brought up. People by now knew we were having issues, and it was hard to confront their faces. Really hard. Vince and Grace had been so sensitive and understated their entire pregnancy, but my brother was hurting. I could tell he was living in the darkness with me. He was struggling with his own feelings. Being a twin, you feel each other's pain in ways that are hard to explain. You are too connected not to. At times, I felt like he wished I could be pregnant instead of them just to relieve me of the pain I was feeling. His sadness was as deep as ours.

Grace, who deserved every moment of indulging in her own pregnancy, was a bit stripped of that attention. But she never seemed to mind, and she always went out of her way to steer the subject away from anything that had to do with pregnancy and kids. The tiptoeing around the subject may not have been fair for her, but I really appreciated it. I just knew I felt good being around them.

On Saturday morning, Jack and I woke up early and escaped to this little coffee shop we loved. It was built into the side of what was built up to look like a huge old-fashioned ship. It overlooked the bay. We got two coffees, mine decaf of course, and took them down to the water to watch the boats sailing in. The morning was perfect—cool and sunny, no humidity. We stared out at the water, thinking. I looked at him and asked, "Remember when you fell off that bouncy floating device in the kiddie pool in Hong Kong?"

"Do I remember? Of course I remember. You laughed at me like a ten-year-old!"

"I was laughing at the face you made as you hung onto the edge so desperately. And at the Chinese kid yelling at you in Hong Kongian."

"Hong Kongian? You know that's not a language, right?"

"Oh, it's a language. Google it."

"I'll Google that glob of blueberry muffin in your tooth first."

"Oh, now you tell me? What kind of husband are you?"

I tried to throw the rest of my coffee on him, but he jetted away too fast. We ran towards the car, knowing that whoever got there first was sure to lock the other one out. Refreshing. All of it. Right down to our sore butts from sitting on the wooden slabs of the bench for an hour. It was a much-needed change from the hustle and bustle of the past few weeks, rekindling a flirt that playfully confirmed the very reasons we married each other in the first place.

We walked back to the house, hand in hand. By the time we

returned, everyone was up. We had breakfast together. The vibe was perfect. It was going to be a good day. I went upstairs to put on my bathing suit. When I looked in the mirror, I remembered all the bruising I had on my lower stomach from the past few months of injections. I was embarrassed to go down to the beach like that. It was a stark reminder of what was going on. We decided to sit up on our roof deck instead. I couldn't wait to get back to the laughs of the morning.

I walked up to the rooftop deck, only to find Grace sitting there with her beautiful little baby bump as well as my cousin's wife, Leah, who was part of the whole Easter pregnancy reveal. She was fully popped as well. I sat there with my cover-up on, mortified about what I was hiding underneath. As time went on and sweat started to gather in the crevices of my body, I knew I had to be brave. I ripped off my cover-up like I was oblivious to the purple blotches underneath.

Maybe no one noticed. Maybe they were good at hiding it. But the shame was burning a hole through my skin, and it was all I could think about. I watched them subtly touch their little swollen bellies and talk about random pregnancy things. Their tone was respectful and low key, and I could handle it. But the chasm between us was obvious. I didn't want them to pity me. I didn't want them to feel bad for me. I just craved for them to understand. I wanted them to somehow appreciate the struggle we were going through to get to a place they had gotten to so easily. That's hard to do unless you have been through it, but I still wanted it.

I heard my brother yell up, "Mike and Anna may be coming to hang."

That news would normally make me excited. Mike and Anna were friends of ours, and I loved a good crew. But Anna was also pregnant, and I immediately panicked, hoping that their plan to swing by would fizzle out. But it didn't, and two hours later, I found myself sitting with three pregnant women and their bellies. As you can imagine, I slipped the cover-up back on.

On top of that, Anna wasn't as aware of what was going on with me, and she kept giggling and chattering to the girls nonstop about being pregnant. Sitting through it was tough. This was supposed to be my day to escape, my weekend to forget, and here I was right smack in the middle of a prenatal summit.

Jack came up to the deck, tapped my shoulder, and quietly reminded me that it was time for the injections. We went downstairs and did them in the bedroom. I pulled up my cover-up. Jack was finding it harder and harder to avoid bruised skin to inject. As he set up the equipment, I heard the girls' laughs coming from the deck. In their carefree voices, I could hear their relief that I had gone. They could finally give free rein to their excitement and happiness. I hated feeling like people were worried about me and holding back because of it. They didn't deserve that either.

Jack gave me the two injections. I think he could tell I was upset, but I saw that he was in a rough place as well. After the shots were done, we sat in silence for a few minutes. He then got up and said he was going to go for a walk. As he left, I remained on the bed. Wishing we were back on the bench laughing about food in my teeth, I stared out into space while the cinema reel playing in my head unspooled all the emotions I was feeling.

Surrounded by people who felt like strangers, I started to cry. I couldn't find anywhere to hide from the reality. My strength had been slowly stripped away as each of those pregnant girls had walked in. I wanted to be stronger than that, but I just couldn't. Jack had taken off, and I was trapped between the swollen telltale face I saw in the mirror and the stork club outside. I didn't want anyone to know I was upset. It wasn't fair to them. It wasn't their fault.

Eventually, my mother came up to check on me. I didn't have to explain a word. The instant she saw my red puffy face, she walked in and closed the door behind her. She hugged me and tried to make me laugh.

"I just feel like everyone around me is pregnant."

She tried to console me, reminding me, "Not everyone. Your cousin Marla isn't pregnant."

I looked up at her, knowing I was about to blow a secret. "She is."

Marla had called that week to tell me. It was still early, and she begged me not to say anything to anyone. Though I appreciated her not isolating me from the news and for telling me in private, it sent me reeling.

My mom stared at me for a second and then her eyes filled with tears. I realized in that moment how hard this process must be for her as well—new territory as a parent, new territory as a friend. Not knowing what to say but being expected to always say the right thing. Whether it was the right thing or the wrong thing, I was glad that she was always there. She was one of the few people who I knew understood and was in the darkness with us. Not that I wanted that for her, but I needed that for me. It was selfish, but it was survival.

I was feeling more and more alone as I traveled further into this journey. People were starting to lose patience with my suffering, moving on with their own lives. I get it. It wasn't their issue. They had their own problems. But their turning away was still hard to bear. I never had a problem that lasted this long—one that took so much time and forbearance. They were moving on, and I was still stuck in place—more alone than ever. I guess I understood. How long were they supposed to comfort me in my disappointment? It was isolating.

Then there was Jack's disappointment as well. My sweet, deep Jack. What must he be thinking? I mean, really feeling. On the outside, he was trying to be supportive, but I could see his heart breaking. He must watch all these girls get pregnant and think why is it so easy for them? The routine was getting old by now. We would get the sad news. I would crumble and cry. He would hug and console me. Then a day later the news would sink in with him, and I would be the one trying to console him. His grief came out differently than mine. Mine poured out in tears. His came with questioning. Sometimes I felt like he was losing hope. It was hard to tell. He had to be thinking about what life would be like if he had married someone younger. He had to be frustrated with me. I consider myself a really nice person, but I know I would be feeling that way if it was his sperm that was the issue. I felt like I couldn't give him the one thing that men dream of their wives giving them. I wanted him to see me with a cute baby belly and wanted him to be proud like the other guys. What was there to be proud of now? I was a disaster of a female—both mentally and physically.

I spent the rest of the weekend passing the time until we could leave. We made up some excuse so that we were able to take off early on Sunday. I just needed to get home. I would try to rebuild once again. We had Dr. Scott and the all-stars in our corner. Our secret weapon. I believed in him. I believed in us. I couldn't lose sight of that.

CHAPTER 20

THE PERKY F%^KING INTERN

My first round with RMA was going smoothly. Their protocols, though a bit different, were basically the same. This round had a positive vibe around it, and I wasn't going to let myself get down. They put me on a steroid as well as the other injections to increase the size of the opening of my uterus. That would help when retrieving the eggs, lessening the chance of damaging any good eggs as they were pulled out. I knew this extra step would work. I knew that the good eggs were just waiting to be found. My little angel was in there somewhere, fighting as hard as I was. Dr. Scott and his dream team were on the case. No yoga pants in this place. These people wore uniforms and legit name tags. They walked in slow motion down the halls to bad ass music and all. They were there to make babies, not for Pilates.

We all know the routine now, right? Injections, blood tests, ultra-sounds for follicle checks, retrieval, fertilization, wait to see if the eggs mature until day six, then send to genetic testing. The injections were going fine, although my beautiful new dining room looked like a pharmacy warehouse with all kinds of syringes and medications from this round and leftovers from the last few. Every time they send you needles, they send you triple of what you need. I guess it's good to have extras, but it was getting harder to find places to store/hide these things. My refrigerator contained beer, milk, and Follistim. I'm just waiting for someone to chug it, thinking it's an energy drink or something. That would be my luck. "IVF patient's thirteen-year-old niece chugs fertility drugs in fridge and gets pregnant with triplets." *Think she'd let me have one?*

When I went in for my first check, I had a little strut to me. I was feeling in control and had full confidence in my team at RMA. I went into the room and started to undress. My underwear was now sitting proudly on a designer pair of flip-flops. Summer's newest IVF fashion, a wonderful sign the seasons had changed from my boots. Such a beautiful image. I was wondering if that underwear would ever see boots again.

Several doctors on Dr. Scott's team were slotted to do the ultrasounds for him. One walked in and introduced himself. He could not be nicer—young looking and so sweet. I didn't know if I wanted to date him or hold him in my arms and rock him to sleep.

He grabbed the wand and began. He counted two follicles.

As much as you think a low number gets easier to hear, it's always so heartbreaking. Again? Was he kidding me? I tried to stay focused. Dr. Scott did say what matters is quality, not quantity, so I had to trust him. By the time I walked out, my strut was gone. I walked down the long hallway, looking in room after room. The blood test room, the ultrasound room, the labs along the hallway. Everyone shared the same look of numbness on their faces. Part scared, part sad, part frustrated, and part sheer nerves while having your blood drawn and awaiting results. You could cut the desperation with a knife. The mundane fears don't go away, and neither do the big ones.

Once inside my car, I made the all-too-customary call to Jack to report that we had just two follicles growing. To finish out the routine, I cried, wiped my nose, composed myself, and went to work. Life doesn't pause for you. Neither does anyone else's. That was a hard reality to swallow as well.

The retrieval went the way I was afraid it would. They retrieved two eggs only. You always hope for a surprise or two, but there was none this time. Both eggs did fertilize, though, and we waited to see if they matured to day six. There was hope in the air. This waiting period was always the hardest. I know that they didn't have many eggs to work with, but I believed in Dr. Scott. Everything that had happened in this round convinced me to keep the faith. I was hoping they would both go for testing, but if it was just one, that would be fine, too. No matter what happened, all the hope in the world wasn't going to change the outcome, so I tried to distract myself for the next six days.

It was only three days later, when as I sat in my office, I looked down at my phone to see that RMA was calling. I thought that was weird. I picked up the phone with a curious hello. There was a voice on the other end that I had never heard before. Almost like a college kid with an airhead voice. She was perky and seemed happy, so I didn't worry too much. "Is this Brett Ruso or Rooso?"

"Yes, this is Brett Russo," I said, emphasizing the correct pronunciation of my name.

She said, "How are you today?"

I'm fine. I'm fine, what did she want? "I'm good."

She went on. "So, your eggs didn't make it past day two."

My heart dropped. That was a first. "They didn't mature at all?"

I felt like a rock was making its way down to my stomach. Before I could say a word, she said, "Nope. You may want to think about an egg donor."

Wait, what? Who was this girl, and why was she giving up on me? What was going on? I was still taking in the bad news. Worst of all, she was so casual.

"Wait, excuse me?" I fired back. "An egg donor? That's what you're suggesting?"

"Well, I don't want to give you false hope that this will work."

"False hope? What do you know about hope? I need to talk to Dr. Scott."

"Well, you'll have to call the call center and make an appointment."

"The call center? Or you could just knock on the wall and get a doctor on the phone!" I was outraged. I was insulted. But most of all, I was frightened. I told myself that she could be an intern and this was her first time she had ever given anyone news. But still. Complete fail. Commoditizing me with her approach.

I hung up the phone. I felt my body starting to shake. I sat there in a void, staring at my computer. I didn't notice how hard my heart was beating. I couldn't breathe. I was having a full-blown anxiety attack. I paged Vince, and he ran in. He tried to calm me down. I knew seeing me cry broke his heart. But I was hysterical. Was this woman kidding me? She was as casual as if she was telling me they were out of the halibut! She had totally given up on me. Did Dr. Scott feel that way? Did Jack feel that way? Was that what everyone was thinking?

I knew I had to get out of there. Vince cleared a path for me to run out without anyone seeing me. I grabbed my bag and ran out of my office. I got to my car and called Jack. I was convulsing and could barely speak. "I'm coming home," he said. I couldn't even tell him not to. I needed him. I needed something.

The car ride back to my house felt like hours. When I finally got home and saw his face, I collapsed in his arms. I unleashed the saddest, most violent cry in all of my life. It was deep and guttural. I don't know what was bothering me more, the fact that the round didn't work or the fact that this nurse had made such an offhand comment. Was I crazy for still believing this whole thing could work? How was this my reality? I felt lost.

Jack tried to console me as I spewed out every thought I was feeling like a frantic lunatic who had officially snapped. He hated to see me cry. I know that he was hurting for me and for himself. His world must have felt like it was spinning. I didn't even ask. I was drowning in my own despair. We were both at a point where we didn't know what to do.

I knew it was time for help. For a while Jack had been suggesting I see a therapist, but I thought I could handle it. Now I knew I couldn't. I went up on the internet and started to Google. I called the first name I could find. Counselor Jenny. She dealt specifically with women and families going through IVF. I called and she picked right up. I couldn't believe it. "This is Counselor Jenny."

I heard her voice on the other end of the line and started to cry again. "I know. I know."

"How soon can you see me?"

"Will next week work?"

Not knowing if I could wait that long, I answered "Yes. That works." I hung up the phone and looked at Jack. "What am I going to do?"

He grabbed me in his arms, and we lay down on the bed. The fact was we had no idea. The appointment was booked, and my life would be on hold until then.

CHAPTER 21

HEAVY EMOTIONAL CONTENT (READER DISCRETION ADVISED)

Do you know what it feels like to lose yourself? I don't mean in the cliché kind of way. I mean to actually feel parts of yourself leaving your body. Parts you loved about yourself. The person you spent a lifetime becoming, slowly floating away. Like you are witnessing your life as it happens, but you aren't inside your own body anymore.

After this last round, I feel like I am desperately fighting to retain anything that I have left of myself. My humor. My positive attitude. My ability to be kind. My ability to control my temperament. My ability to be social. And my ability to see the purpose of it all. I feel it all slipping away, and I don't know how to stop it. The harder I try to be the person I used to be, the less genuine it feels. Maybe this

IVF process changes you forever. Maybe trying to reinvent yourself is part of what makes you one of those people everyone talks about that "rose above" and was so strong and positive. I want to be that person, but I don't know her anymore. The stakes have gotten too high, and I'm in way further than I ever thought I'd be. The disappointments are too real. And the darkness is too deep. I don't feel equipped to handle this.

Summer has come, and all I want to do is be that light-hearted girl I used to be, but I don't have it in me. She's lost. I am trying to find her again. I miss her. I miss her passion for bringing people together. I miss her ability to bring out the best in people. I have started to feel like I don't have what it takes to rise above anymore. Who am I trying to be anyway? I hope she is not lost forever. I don't know if people understand what a roller-coaster this is. I know that it's "not cancer," and I know it doesn't seem difficult for people who aren't going through it. But it is so emotionally draining. The all-encompassing ups and downs. The managing the expectations of the people around you. Defending yourself in order to salvage any hope you have left. It is constant. The feelings are constant. Though you can forget about them for a while, they always swing back. Keeping them away has become exhausting.

We went down to the shore the next weekend with all of Jack's friends from college. The time away was supposed to make me forget. But all it did was make me realize how far behind everyone else I was. Hearing other mothers talk about their children and share parenting stories was so hard. I couldn't relate, nor did I care. I watched their mouths move, but all I could think was, *Why isn't this us? Why don't we deserve it?* I used to be the woman who played with other people's children. A year ago, I would have been. But that weekend I couldn't muster up the stamina or the interest. What kind of mother would I even be right now anyway? I felt like I hated their kids. What kind of mother hates kids?

I got cornered by one of my friend's wives. She was drunk and, well, kind of an asshole to start. I had met her that night. We were having a BBQ with about thirty of Jack's friends and their wives and kids. It was dinnertime all of a sudden, and as you can imagine, the rush to get the food on the table was crazy. I went into the garage to get more paper plates. As I was fishing around in obscure beach cabinets, the kind that contain both beach paddles and toilet paper—she came in and cornered me.

She said, "I'm so sorry about the baby."

I had no idea what she was talking about, nor did I realize she knew about our situation. I assumed she meant IVF and just said, "Oh, thank you." Then she went on and on about her friend who had a miscarriage.

I said to her, "You may think I'm someone else. I didn't have a miscarriage."

She said immediately, "You didn't? I thought you went through IVF?"

I said, "Well, I did. Three rounds actually, but it didn't work."

Her eyes widened, and in a loud voice as if I just told her a story of a mass murder I committed or something, "It didn't work? WHY!"

Please walk away. Oh God, please walk away. You don't know what you are doing to me right now. Have you ever had to explain IVF to someone who has no clue—someone who had four kids by the time she was thirty? You don't even know where to start. I started fumbling and saying, "Well, we had three embryos, but they weren't genetically sound."

"What do you mean!?" I just couldn't explain. Oblivious, she said, "I'm sorry. By the way, I don't eat meat. Do you happen to have a little pasta we can make?"

Everything had gone in one ear and out the other. It was as if I was talking to Dory in *Finding Nemo*. I guess I was relieved that she changed the subject. It also made me realize how scarily insignificant my life was to everyone else. I was officially inside every girl's nightmare. This was my reality, and there was no off switch.

A few days later, we went in to see Dr. Scott. I took him up on his promise to always be honest with me and asked him for the truth. He explained to me that based on my statistics, four unsuccessful rounds—we had now gone through three—could be a strong indicator that this process may not work for us. He added that I was a perfect candidate for an egg donor. Hearing the words come out of his mouth felt more real than when Miss *Legally Blonde* intern said them. It was easier to hear, though not necessarily easier to swallow. Everything made more sense coming from him, and I trusted him.

So much was riding on this last round, and that was a very scary thought. I have always wanted children. I wanted to see myself in my child. I wanted to see the qualities that I have in this little person. That was an important part of it for me. If I had to use an egg donor, I knew I would accept it eventually, but I was far from mentally being ready to deal with that. I couldn't believe that we were already looking that decision in the face.

The part that was really starting to mess with my head was the mind-over-matter versus the scientific facts. My nature is to be positive, and that has always made me succeed. If work is slow, I work my ass off and bring more sales in. Presto! Not slow anymore. If I'm playing a sport and we are down, I rally the team and play with all my heart. Voilà! We win. That attitude has always made me come out on top.

IVF, though—this is different. This is cold science. No change in thinking and no amount of hard work would affect the outcome. No matter how positively I think, I couldn't will the outcome. On the contrary, positive thinking only became a source of built-up disappointment. Hope had become a bad word in my house. It's like I was doing something wrong when I said things like, *"This is it"* or *"I have a good feeling about this one."* It felt like I was being a fool. The mental drop from positivity to disappointment was a long fall.

And where does God fit into all of this? I see the abyss in the ground in front of me, and it's taking every bone in my body not to fall in. But it doesn't go away. It's always there. These new feelings are foreign to me, and I don't know how to adjust to them. It's as if the world is speaking in a new language and I don't know how to communicate. Especially at night. When I go to bed, I stare at the dresser in the corner of my room. It's like a TV screen that plays this nightmare I'm living in over and over—disbelief that this is my life, unfamiliar with the grief I'm feeling, visions of holding my child in my arms. Things I want so badly but are not within my reach. All I can do is sit and wait. I can't try harder. I can't do any more. I am in over my head. All I know is I need to make it to that therapy appointment.

CHAPTER 22

COUNSELOR JENNY

I turned into the driveway of a small house with Counselor Jenny's name outside. Seeing a parking lot in the back, I pulled in and waited. I was early for my appointment. A part of me felt like starting the car right up again and driving away. I was feeling a little better after last week's trauma and thought maybe I didn't need this after all. I almost felt goofy being there. I'd never seen a therapist in my life. What was she going to tell me that I couldn't tell myself? I kept checking the clock and then my email, looking for any excuse not to go in. With ten minutes to go, I decided to go for it and walked in. Brett Russo, officially in therapy. This should be interesting.

I walked into what once was obviously an old living room. It smelled a little musty, and it didn't look all that professional—but it was quaint. It was calming in an *after midnight the ghosts in this house will kill you* sort of way. As soon as I sat on the couch, I heard her come down the hall. Counselor Jenny was shorter than I imagined. Younger than I expected. Sweet-looking. She called my name as if there were six other people in the waiting room. I looked around, confirming there were no other patients and answered, "Yes, that's me."

Her office had everything you would expect in a therapist's room. A couch for me, a seat for her, tissues, a lamp, some books, and a notepad on which she could write down how messed up I was. I sat on the couch and adjusted my skirt a little. She gazed at me, expecting me to open up. Yet I didn't know how to start or how to describe to her who I was. How would she know how to deal with my feelings if she didn't know what kind of person I was? Would my outfit give her clues? Was she reading my behavior already?

I decided to beat her to the awkward first words to show her I was cool and collected, "So...I guess I should start by..." and then I started sobbing.

Without any warning, tears started pouring from my eyes. She handed me a tissue. "I just don't know how I got here." I could barely speak as I cried even harder. All I could think about was how a short while ago I was in Hawaii gleefully planning our family to the tunes of the ocean breeze, and now, I'm sitting in a shrink's office talking about adopting eggs from strangers.

Her silence wasn't helping. Was she even a shrink? The sign said counselor. What does that even mean? Is that a lesser degree than a psychologist? Is that like a peer minister you used to have in high school? Do you even need to go to college for that? Plus, she looked younger than me, and that made me skeptical as well.

"I know, Brett. I know." Her eyes were filling with tears, too. "I have two children. My first was through IVF and my second was through an egg donor. All I can tell you is that I love both these children fiercely, and neither means more to me than the other. I know that you're in a world of pain. I wish I could tell you the pain goes away. But it doesn't. This process will change you. But you will see that you will be better for it if you let yourself."

Hearing those words come out of her mouth humanized her. We were the same in a lot of ways. I realized that this thing is always a part of you and the mourning that you feel never really goes away. I started to open up to her about things I was feeling. I found talking to her was easy because I didn't feel guilty letting out what I had been feeling. I spoke about how hard it was when people that had miscarriages thought they knew what I was going through. We talked about how hard it was to see the people around me starting families so easily. We talked about Jack and me and how much I felt at fault. She told me how important it was to communicate and make sure that we were speaking our minds to each other: good, bad, or ugly. She just seemed to get it, even in that short time of talking with her. We were really connecting. I really felt like we were getting somewhere together. We got into some pretty deep shit. The possibilities of this newfound friendship felt endless. Who knew what would come next? Lunches, dinners? Facebook friends?

Then she abruptly announced that our time was up. I was like wait, what? *What was all that "one in a million" talk?* We made so much headway! I thought we were friends! I found myself wanting to stay. I immediately told her that I wanted to come back.

We set up an appointment for the following week. She stood up over me as if to say, *Don't let the door hit you on the way out.* I stood up. I got that she had a role to play. Now do I hug her? Was that a thing? I had never hugged my doctor before. But she's a counselor. Can you hug counselors? We had just shared so much.

I walked out the door, turned around, and went in for the hug. She was fine with it...*ish.* But I didn't care. I walked down the hall. I turned around right before I went down the stairs, expecting to see her look back at me again, as if to say, "You've got this, girl." But all I saw was her door closing. She was on to crazy patient 3:30 p.m.

While our hour might have been merely another session to her, it meant the world to me. I walked out of there feeling revived—not because she listened to my story, but because I listened to hers. She had once been in my shoes, and she had come out on the other side. Hearing her talk, seeing her tear up, and feeling her connect so closely with the emotions I was feeling made me realize that I could find hope in the fact that women had braved this journey before me. I was not a victim this was happening to; I was someone who was going to fight her way through. Like her. Like the me I knew I could be.

I had to keep holding out hope in the vision that a light was waiting for me at the end of the tunnel. I just had to get there. A happy outcome on the other side of this was beckoning to me. I just had to be patient and not write my ending before it happened. I was an IVF patient, and like her, I was not going to let failure triumph.

CHAPTER 23

TJ MAXX

The house was coming along great. We were becoming more and more settled in our new suburban life. Though I couldn't get a manicure or a decent salad after seven, I was starting to relax into all the peaceful aspects it did offer—like chipmunks running across the porch and dinners we grilled outside. I found myself obsessed with decorating, and by now, the entire downstairs was set up. Maybe it was my way of distracting myself. But all my free time was spent on Amazon or in TJ Maxx.

The house had four beautiful bedrooms upstairs, all painted different colors. One had all our old NYC furniture. It looked like a little in-law suite. The others were bare except for random pieces of furniture from the owner before. The possibilities were endless, and I found myself consumed with thoughts about what theme to make each bedroom. I needed to feel settled. I needed to feel like the house was neat and ready to live in.

I can't describe what made me so restless, but it became like a sickness. I wanted Jack to feel at home. This was going to be a place where our friends and family would visit. It was supposed to represent a place that was good and pure, and happy. Every time I walked past these rooms I was haunted by their emptiness. Their lack of soul. As if they represented the life we couldn't quite have.

The first TJ Maxx run targeted the "blue room." My mom and I spent hours in the store finding the perfect knickknacks to complete our nautical theme. We bought bedding and then backup bedding for that bedding. We bought a huge stuffed whale and this fake vintage bocce ball bag that looked like it was stolen right out of the Kennedy compound for the corner of the room. There was a built-in desk in another corner. I filled a little copper cup with pencils. I even bought a sharpener and sharpened each one. I placed one of those old composition notebooks next to the bed with a little pen on top as if someone had been writing in it and then decided to put it down and go to bed. The finished project was perfect. Like a little dollhouse.

The second room was already painted a pale yellow. It had a bed as well as a flowered nightstand. Twelve hundred dollars in bedding later, it looked like a little girl's flowered paradise. This room was probably my least favorite, but the look was good for now. Someday, it would be the obvious choice for a nursery, so I didn't want to take the decor too far.

The last room was very wide, perfect for two beds. I pictured two twin girls telling each other their secrets all night or a guest room that all our friends would fight over. I went online and bought two queen-size mattresses, box springs, and bed frames. I found a farm in the Midwest that made custom headboards, and I bought a natural wood headboard for each bed. I didn't tell Jack about this room. I wanted him to come home one night and see what I had done. This room screamed "Scandinavian ski house" to me.

Back to TJ Maxx I went. I bought moose heads and tribal-looking decorative balls. I discovered a collection of wooden bowls that looked like there were trees coming out of the tops, an arrangement of fake branches that looked like hiking sticks all wrapped together, and two Alpaca ottomans that were perfect for the window alcove. I bought a huge oversized chair with a plaid blanket thrown over it. It looked like a ski house in the Alps.

This was the room I was most excited about. Jack rarely went upstairs. *Wait until he saw this one*, I kept thinking. As I added the finishing touches, I couldn't wait for him to come home from work.

I jumped in the shower. I felt good. I was starting to feel settled. I was proud of what I had done, what we had weathered so far. The words of Counselor Jenny kept echoing in my head, and I felt inspired. I decided in that moment that I was not giving up. It was as if someone took a machine and started pumping conviction back into my body. I had this overwhelming feeling that there were eggs inside of me—healthy little eggs, and I had to find them. I was not going to stop fighting. I couldn't wait to see Jack. I know he had missed the old Brett—the one who was energetic, happy, and positive. I felt "back." I got out of the shower, put on a cute sundress, and awaited Jack's arrival.

When he walked into the house, I had a pep to my step as I skipped up to greet him. I told him I had a surprise for him. He looked intrigued. I brought him upstairs, and his face became even more perplexed. He smirked, not knowing what to expect. I walked into the room ahead of him because I wanted to see his reaction.

I opened the door: "Tada…" He looked into the room and his face went blank. Was he in shock? Was he overwhelmed with excitement and so impressed that he didn't know how to react? He said, "Wow, this is…" he paused, "a lot of beds." He just stood in the doorway without moving. "I thought we were going to make this a gym or a playroom."

I was appalled with his response. The room was perfect for a two-bed bedroom. It was made for that. "Do you not like it?"

"No, I like it. It's really…really…" He then left the room.

I was picking up a weird vibe. I followed him down the hall, "Are you sure you like it? I thought we discussed that this would be a good room for two beds."

"I like it. Really."

I was probably being oversensitive. The poor guy had just walked in from one of his treacherous commutes. I needed to give him some time to digest his excitement.

He went downstairs, and I followed him down. He had brought home some takeout Thai food for us. I set the table, and we sat down. Before we could take our first bite, I announced, "I'm not giving up. I decided today, babe. I don't care how many rounds it takes. I don't care what it does to me. I know that our baby is in there, and I am not going to give up."

He didn't seem moved by my conviction. "Well, you can't do this forever."

I was stopped dead in my victory lap. What did he mean? Was he telling me that he was ready to give up? Did he think I was crazy for thinking this way? Was he starting to get frustrated with me and all the failures? Did he not like the Scandinavian theme? I thought he would be so inspired to hear me talk like this.

Maybe we were on different pages. A new barrage of questions exploded in my head. Did I ever take the time to ask him how he was feeling? Did I even care? Did he still *want* children?

"And what is with all the rooms?" he said. "I thought that we would decorate them as we go. I thought that we would use them for our family someday." He had an aggression to his voice that I had never heard before. "Who are we right now?"

I got very defensive. "You don't like the rooms? I have literally been working on them for weeks. This is information you could've told me earlier!"

"Well, I just thought that we would decorate them together with things we got from the places we've actually been and will go. Not this. What is this? I don't even know what this is."

He went on and on. I didn't know how to unhear some of the

things he was saying, fighting how hurtful it felt, knowing how right he was.

I felt so small. I had never heard that tone in his voice before, especially not directed at me. I felt insulted. I felt sad. I felt stupid. I felt embarrassed. But worst of all, I felt so bad that he felt this way, and I didn't take the time to notice. I fired back with some hugely defensive rant about pencils and bedding, knowing full well that it had nothing to do with any of that at all.

Once the yelling stopped, we sat in silence, staring at our dishes. I didn't know what to say. I didn't know how we were going to get past everything we had just said to each other. We had never really had a fight before. I didn't know that was coiled inside us. How could we have gotten so far down this path without knowing how each of us was feeling? I was held captive by the awkwardness, with nowhere to look but down.

Jack walked toward the sink with his half-filled plate, saying he wasn't hungry.

As he walked out, I said the only thing that came to my mind. "Well, Counselor Jenny says that it's always better to say what's on your mind, even if it may hurt the other person's feelings."

He turned around, looked at me, and started to laugh. He came back toward me and me toward him. Meeting in the middle, we hugged. And I cried. And we hugged harder. And I cried harder.

The episode opened the door to the most real, raw, and important conversation we had ever had. I realized that my obsession with decorating those rooms was because it broke my heart to see them empty. But it broke his to see them filled for people that didn't exist. I realized that his realism and my optimism had to meet in the middle. We had no other choice but to start thinking through all our options. An egg donor was the unspoken elephant in the room.

I've come to learn that this process is tougher on a marriage than I ever imagined. It's scary because the aftereffects run deeper than making up after a typical fight. You don't realize you aren't communicating because both of you are in protection mode. You want to protect yourself and protect your partner. You may not even realize that changes are taking place. The drifting apart is very subtle, and if you don't address it, the effects can be fatal to the relationship. When I consider couples I know who argue about issues that are so less important, I often wonder how they would handle IVF. Would they even know how to? Would they survive?

I was proud of us. Even though it was a tough night and what he said was eye opening, baring our feelings was healthy. I felt a little lighter because of it.

The next morning, I waited for Jack to leave for work. When I heard his car turn out of the driveway, I went upstairs with a big black garbage bag and started to throw away all the meaningless knickknacks that filled those rooms with fake memories—memories that weren't ours. Memories that were manufactured. Souvenirs of trips that we never took. With each new object I put into the bag, I felt more and more silly. The pencils that no one had ever used. The empty notebooks on the desk. Wooden tribal bowls from the African safari we never took that still had TJ Maxx stickers attached to the bottom.

Each room's display was stupid and unauthentic. I felt embarrassed. I found myself at an important turning point. I kept only a few of the items. The rooms looked slightly bare, but that was okay.

Jack was right. Our family story was not yet written, and we didn't have to make it something it wasn't. We would get there. Life was starting to stray off the straight track, and we were going to have to learn to do the same, together. I dragged the garbage bag into a back closet and closed the door. It was a story not written yet, one that couldn't be bought. It was time to start facing some realities.

♪ CHAPTER 24 ♪

DONOR? I DON'T EVEN KNOW 'ER!

With the big TJ Maxx fight behind us, it was time to start exploring all our options. The choices included everything from acupuncture to eating pineapples. Theories on ways to get pregnant were everywhere you turned. Some advocated a gluten-free/dairy-free diet. Some said eat rare meat. Some swore by all types of vitamins that claimed to help with egg quality.

Doing research also meant learning more about the egg donor process. Each day that passed, I tried my best to become more comfortable with that thought. But it was hard. Really hard. I felt like another woman's egg would make everyone else feel better: Jack would have his kid. The people around me would be able to put the drama of my getting pregnant to bed. Everyone would get what they wanted. Everyone but me. The closer I got to saying I would accept it, the further I felt mentally.

That week, I met with Counselor Jenny. This time I was fully prepared with a list of issues I wanted to talk about, especially now that I knew she'd turn off our session, and our "friendship," the second that little buzzer rang. She'd said that she had a son through an egg donor, and I wanted to learn more about this. The thought felt so foreign to me. Even the words coming out of my mouth didn't feel like my own. But I knew it would be a process and learning more would be the start. People were counting on me to get there emotionally. I was starting to feel the pressure looming over me.

"How did you know you were ready?" I asked her.

"I remember the day. I woke up, and I was done. Done with the needles. Done with the heartbreak. I just knew I was ready to be a mom again."

"Where do you even begin?"

"There are many different options. You can go on a waiting list for live donors, which can take time. Or you can go to an egg bank, where you can purchase eggs that are frozen. You literally get a stack of resumes, like you're on a dating site that tell you all about the mother and everything she's done. Sometimes they include personal letters. Sometimes pictures. You can search for someone who fits you and pick qualities that are important to you as a couple."

While she was in the middle of her explanation, I looked down, covered my face with my hand, and started to cry. She touched my arm.

"This is not easy to accept. You have to go through a mourning process first, mourning the loss of the ability to have a baby the way you always dreamed you would. What you're feeling is normal. But I promise you this: That baby will feel no less yours. That I can promise you."

I felt guilty for crying over a procedure she had already gone through. I didn't want her to think I was being insensitive, nor did I want her to think that I looked down on her or her family. The idea was just so hard to swallow. She went on to tell me that certain forms of DNA, called mitochondrial RNA, are transferred from the carrier to the baby, so the baby can inherit traits of the mother who carries the pregnancy. At first, it felt like a phony clinical finding, a consolation prize that someone made up to make women feel better. After discussing it further with Dr. Scott, though, I found out that the phenomenon was real. It made me feel less like a human incubator and more like a mother.

When I got home that night, I talked to Jack about all the things Counselor Jenny and I had discussed about the egg donor process. He was happy and almost relieved that I was making an attempt to wrap my head around the concept. "So, you get to pick out a donor from hundreds of profiles. It's actually much more personal than you would think."

He was really into it. "So, we could drink wine and sit by the fire and pick our family. It would be awesome," he said as he smiled.

"Totally! And we can invite our friends over and make a party around it."

"Yeah and then we can get a tall blonde or a Harvard grad or something like that as a donor."

I stopped short in disbelief. "No, asshole, the point is that you get someone like ME! Someone who hates to read! A little brunette with no boobs and a big ass! Someone who played field hockey and loves Christmas."

"Blondes like Christmas! I'm kidding. I'm kidding!"

Yeah, he was kidding. Just as much as I was kidding about having a party around picking our egg donor. The prospect of it suddenly had a weird effect on me, and I didn't want to talk about it anymore. I realized that on the surface I was trying to go along, but on the inside, I was further away than ever.

So, what did I do? I made an acupuncture appointment and bought three pineapples. This fight wasn't over.

⚰ CHAPTER 25 ⚱

A BABY SHOWER

I had an anxiety attack in the shower. I almost passed out. I had to yell for Jack at 6:30 a.m., covered in soap and shampoo. My chest felt like it was closing, and I couldn't breathe. I ran out of the shower the best I could and climbed back into bed. Jack covered my soaking wet body in blankets and held me. He tried to talk through what I was feeling as I stayed focused on taking deep breaths, the empty shower still running behind me. I felt like a shell of a woman, lying there naked. My body giving in. My mind losing the fight. My heart too waterlogged to move.

I feel like I'm in the middle of a shit storm. I've started to have trouble sleeping. If I'm alone with my thoughts too long, darkness settles in. Panic. The reality that IVF may not work for us. A lot is riding on this round, but I don't feel pressure, as there's nothing I can really do to affect the outcome. I feel myself wanting to pray or have faith in something, but I don't know what that means or who that means. Is it God? Is it karma? Is it Mother Nature? Or is it just that the outcome is what's meant to be, and I have to find peace in that? All I can do is wait. Hope for the best, expect the worst?

Hope continues to be a weird thing. Everyone expects me to have it, but when it crashes in my face, no one is there to see me cry. I almost feel guilty when I feel hopeful. Where does that come from? And why? Why on top of everything else do I have to feel guilty about trying to be positive?

I know I've been dark. I hate that you have to see me like this. I want to be inspirational. I want to tell you that it's gotten better. But I can't. I want to tell you that it will get better. But I can't. I know these thoughts have been heavy. But I just can't find the humor in anything anymore. It's getting too serious. Before it was, "Well, this is the route we have to take. It sucks, but the end result will be the same." Now I am starting to wonder what that end result will be. Does it mean nothing and I keep living my life the way I have for the past thirty-eight years? Am I doomed to be the barren old aunt who never had children of her own?

My life has become a cycle of feeling down, picking myself up, being there for a hot second, and then getting news that brings me back down again. It's as if someone for whatever reason doesn't want me to feel hopeful for too long. Or at peace. Or just normal for a goddamned second. I miss myself more than you could ever know. I don't know how to get her back until I'm through all of this. She doesn't fit into this world I'm living in now. It's cold and dark. It's a frightening place to be. It's almost like I want to protect her from this so that she can come back as the same naively happy girl that I left behind. Counselor Jenny says that this process changes you. That I'm fighting to be the same person who I was before all of this,

but I'm not the same person anymore. I'm changed. And that's okay.
But is it okay? What if I didn't want to change? What if I liked me
the way I was?

Today was a rough day. On top of starting the injections for Round Four—the "last shot" in the implied words of Dr. Scott—I had to attend my cousin Leah's baby shower. I didn't want to go, but I knew I should. It was just always hard for me—hard seeing what I wanted so badly right smack in front of me, wondering what people were thinking, worrying about what they were going to ask.

It was a really hot day. I was about ten pounds overweight, which is a lot when you're five-foot-two. I slicked my hair back in a tight bun and started the process of finding something to wear. My room looked like a bomb hit it when I was done. I finally narrowed it down to a pretty flowery sundress. It looked a little Hawaiian for my typical taste, but it felt happy. It also grazed over most of my thigh fat and bloated stomach, so it was definitely my most slimming option. It didn't do much for my extra chin, but nothing was going to fix that. *Jack, does this dress make my face look fat?* All in all, I felt good.

Leah lived about an hour's drive from my house. I was late to begin with as I debated whether to say I was sick and ditch the whole thing. By the time I pulled in and parked my car, the long curb was filled with cars I recognized. I grabbed my gift from the back seat and headed up the steep driveway. When I finally made it to the top, I was sweating and panting. This from a former Division One athlete, mind you. Unreal. Anyway, I walked in the door and all the guests were seated facing in my direction. Everyone stared at me. I looked around the room and caught my mother's eye. She looked like a deer in the headlights.

I didn't quite understand until I looked to my right. There, to my horror, I saw the same pink Hawaiian flowery pattern I was wearing. At first, I thought I was looking in a mirror, but it was Leah, poised to begin opening her gifts. We were wearing the same exact dress. Only difference was she was seven months pregnant. And, for the record, "wore it best." I was mortified.

I had no choice but to hug her and laugh on the outside while everyone snapped pictures of the "hysterical" coincidence, but on the inside, I wanted to crawl into a ball and die. I made my way around the room saying my hellos. Everyone was looking down at my stomach. Wondering. Wanting to ask the question. Assuming by my lack of a neck and the maternity dress I was wearing that I was probably pregnant. That was always the worst part about being in cycle. I was swollen and not drinking, so observers watching closely naturally thought I was pregnant when, ironically, I was as far from it as possible.

I finally made my way to my mother and my other cousins. They spoke over each other as if to change the subject and to ask questions about the new house and make me laugh. But someone might as well have turned off the sound in the room because all I could hear was what they were thinking. Their pity. I stayed for an hour and then said I had to go. As I was leaving, a few more people begged me to wait so that they could take a picture of Leah and me together. How funny were we in the same dress? She's pregnant, and she's not. Yeah. Hysterical. I smiled on the outside, though I wanted to vanish into thin air.

I felt taunted by the world. I made it home with enough time to recover before my evening injections. Another attempted day, another battle lost—wasted sadness taking the place of an occasion that should've been happy. Time that should've been spent celebrating the most important people in my life had been hijacked by my selfish feelings of self-pity. It's time I will never get back.

It's times like this you need to dig deep. Your inner darkness wants to test you. You need to count on the people in your life to make you whole again. I know it's easier said than done. Maybe I am convincing myself by writing this. But one thing I've learned is that if I give up, then the end is here. I wasn't ready for this to be my ending, and I especially refused to go down in a Hawaiian dress.

CHAPTER 26

A WITCH'S TIT

On a cool fall Sunday morning, one of the first of the season, the sun had just risen over the horizon, and a low mist hovered over the fields of hay along the road. The air had that festive, haunting October feeling. I was on my way for my first follicle check of this next round. Round Four. With barely any cars on the road, I felt a peace in the air, as if the world was opening up to feed my soul before my blood test. These early morning appointments belonged to me.

At this point in the round, you have to go back every few days for your blood tests and follicle checks. You could go anytime between six and ten in the morning, but I chose the early mornings because they had a calming effect. I could soak in the results before I had to face anyone. Time was standing still for me alone. It was a time in which I could regain a piece of my old self. Jack always offered to come with me but going alone was therapeutic. It gave me a chance to work through the before and after of whatever result the morning would bring.

On the way there, I was always hopeful as I tried to reconnect with the warrior inside me. But like clockwork, the ride home left me feeling like a prisoner again, captured by disappointing news, held hostage by the car door as I often lingered inside long after the engine had stopped to shield Jack from whatever result had been revealed. I needed time to work through how I would tell him, time to work through how I would tell myself.

The waiting room was crowded for a Sunday morning—as if the building was a time warp where life never stopped inside, not even to sleep. The nurses were all talking casually about their weekends. This was just a job to them. I wondered if they had any idea the mountain of pain in the hearts of the women who sat in those chairs day in and day out, feeling an ache that went so far deeper than the prick of their needles.

As I waited for my blood work, I put my hand in my jacket pocket. I felt a crumbled piece of paper at the bottom. Curious, I pulled it out. It was my NYCM name tag from the winter before. I couldn't believe that I was on the second season of this winter jacket, still getting infertility blood tests. It was a hopeless feeling, as if the world was moving forward around me, yet I was frozen in time. I stared at the paper in my hand, crinkled and stained. As much as I hated it, I couldn't throw it away. It represented a deeper struggle for me now. I placed it back in my pocket when a nurse calling my name snapped me back into reality.

I walked into the ultrasound room. My body was shaking, but the room wasn't cold. I was tired. I was scared. I felt defeated. I was desperate to know what this round would bring. It felt like I was watching a tree fall in slow motion from above me but was unable to move out of its way.

The doctor walked in and greeted me with a warm smile. I liked this particular doctor. She had a kindness in her eyes. She looked younger than she probably was, and she always made me feel relaxed. I leaned back on the table and closed my eyes. I couldn't look at the screen. The sad truth was, with three rounds behind me, I knew what to look for, and I couldn't bear a low number again.

Then she started counting under her breath. Two, three, five, six...my heart skipped a beat. Was I hearing correctly? Was she counting follicles? I didn't see sheep in the room! Was she looking inside the right vagina? It was only the first check, I reminded myself. Still, I sat up and looked at her as she pulled the wand out.

She went back to her chart and said, "Okay, we'll see you back in three days."

"Wait, doc, what did you find?"

"You have ten follicles growing."

I stared at her in disbelief, adrenaline pumping through my entire body.

"It's still early, but that's a great start."

No shit and a witch's tit, it was a good start! I had NEVER had that many.

She left the room, and I found myself pacing, not knowing what to do. I was breathing hard and laughing and tearing up, saying, "Oh my God" to myself over and over. I had to get home to tell Jack.

I grabbed my underwear from my shoe, hopping on one foot, tripping toward the door. But I found my balance. Not today, underwear! Not today!

I was no dummy. I knew it was early, and anything could happen, but in that one festive October moment, I felt I had stolen back a piece of my own happiness. I felt alive, and I had to enjoy it. Who knew how long it would last?

Back home, I pulled into the driveway and had barely shut off the car before I found myself halfway in the door. I ran to the bedroom. Jack was still in bed but heard me as I stumbled in.

I screamed, "We have ten follicles growing! We have ten, ten, ten follicles growwwwing!"

He looked at me with his eyes wide and smiling as if he didn't believe it. "Okay, okay, let's not get ahead of ourselves," he said, nervous as he always was for me when I got my hopes up.

But his warning was too late. My hopes were so high that they could float away, and it felt amazing. "Oh, you mean stop decorating the nursery? I thought a sea salt gray for the walls would be best!"

"Come on now. Just calm down." He gave me a look like he was going to scold me. "Everyone knows pale yellow works better."

His joke made me realize that he wanted to play along, too. More cautious than me but showing glimmers of hope. Maybe this was it. Maybe it wasn't. I didn't care. All I knew was that the good news felt glorious.

I was scheduled to go back three days later to see how the follicles were growing. I couldn't wait. My entire mentality changed. I felt hopeful, I felt energized, and I felt like it was finally my turn. Good news makes you erase all the bad news in an instant. It's crazy how your brain can do that. As if it wants to forget all the trauma that went before. With ten follicles growing, the possibilities were endless. Maybe I could have more than one child, after all. I went back to thoughts of twins and family Christmases dancing in my head.

The days went by so slowly. I started to open up to people. I finally had a story of success to tell. I was on my way to leaving all this behind me. I even found myself telling my drycleaner that I was going through IVF and that I just had some really good results. As if she cared or knew what I was talking about. She did respond with, "Oh, I could tell by the blood on your shirts." So yeah, okay, that was a weird response, especially since I had never heard her speak before but who cares? I was about to have kids!

For the next appointment I arrived twenty minutes before the door even opened. I waited as the doctors and nurses filed in. I watched them hang up their coats and put their lunches in the fridge, making small talk along the way with each other. I tried to distract myself, but I was too anxious.

When they called me into the room, I was sweating. You know

that feeling you get as you are slowly riding up to the top of the biggest dip on the roller coaster? I took off my shoes and socks, rolled up my pants to my knees and sat on the high table.

When the doctor walked in, she said, "Okay, I'll need you to remove your slacks."

I looked at her, confused, and then I realized that in my happy delirium I had prepared my pants for a pedicure, not an ultrasound. My brain was spazzing all over the place. It was embarrassing and funny all at the same time. Neither feeling distracted me from the results that were so close to being revealed. I took off my slacks and sat up on the table again.

The doctor searched the screen. On it I saw two large follicles as she moved the wand around. Sometimes it's hard to tell if you are looking at new follicles or the same ones over and over again. Where is a damn medical degree when you need one? I kept seeing these two big ones come up. It seemed like the same ones, but I couldn't tell. She then checked the other side, which seemed to have no action. That wasn't totally uncommon.

She removed the wand and said I could sit up. "I see two follicles." Only two? Not this game again.

"What do you mean? There were ten last time we checked."

She explained that I had two decent-sized follicles growing at a nice, equal pace. She'd found a few other small ones, but there was little action. In one deflating moment, I was back to where we started.

As she left the room, my body weighed me down so heavily on the table that it felt like I could fall through it. It was happening again. Desperation. I knew the feeling all too well. I didn't think I would be returning to that state. Falling from my dreams into a nightmare once again.

I called Jack from the room, but he didn't answer. I pulled the collar of my jacket up as far as it could go to hide my face and walked quickly to escape that place before I completely lost it. As I got to my car, I felt my phone vibrating from my bag. It was time to tell Jack the news. What would he say? I would have to tell him that he was right about getting my hopes up too high. I was a foolish girl. Who was I to think otherwise?

I picked up the phone, surprised to hear the voice on the other end. It was my brother. Grace was in labor.

CHAPTER 27

PERFECT

The parking garage of the hospital where Grace and Vince were having the baby was filled with cars of all sizes. It was raining, and everyone must have been using the lot to keep dry. As I drove through the bottom level, I saw that most of the spots were empty, but they were reserved for hospital personnel, handicapped stickers, and of course "Expectant Mothers." The thought occurred to me: how would they know I wasn't expecting? They certainly can't give you an ultrasound right there in the parking lot. My luck I would be stopped by the security guard, saying, "I'm sorry, miss, I don't really see that pregnancy glow."

I kept driving. The cement ramp took me in twists and turns from level to level as the place was filled to capacity. Every time I made a turn, my wet tires would make this loud gut-wrenching squeak. As if I needed new brakes. The kind of noise that you want to tell people immediately, it's not my fault! Each screeching turn, higher and higher in the lot, was a harsh reminder that I was heading farther and farther from those expectant mother spots.

The annoyance of it started to bristle under my skin. I finally found a spot on the top level—the only level without a roof. I took a deep breath, opened the door, and ran for cover.

When I opened the door to the maternity waiting room, I saw familiar faces everywhere, both from our side of the family and Grace's. On a small coffee table in the middle of the room, my mother had set out a buffet of pastries, cookies, and baby decorations. She had a bag filled with crossword puzzles and magazines. She was obviously expecting a long wait. Grace's parents were much quieter, and I could tell they were nervous for their daughter.

I tried to picture my brother in the delivery room. Was he scared? Was he excited? Did he need me? He was about to meet this little person who would become the main focus in his life. Would he still have time for me? Would he remember me? Was this the end of life as I knew it?

With each passing minute, new people arrived. Some cousins, Grace's sister, and her boyfriend. My older brother and his wife. Positive energy filled the air as everyone was anxiously waiting for an update from within. At 10:00 a.m., Grace's sister got the first text from them: "Contractions pretty intense, but they just gave Grace an epidural." Her sister jumped out of her chair with nerves and excitement as she read it out loud. But all I could think was why didn't I get a text? I kept looking at my phone waiting for my text from Vince. But it didn't appear. Had he forgotten about me already? Grace's sister got a text, and I'm sure they love each other, but, well, I'm the twin. I'm different. Was there no room left for me in his thoughts? Was he with his new family now and my lack thereof was not an issue he would have time for anymore?

Then my phone lit up. And then again, and again. "It's happening. Stinky, it's happening."

"So far so good"..."Contractions are getting stronger. Epidural soon"..."How you holding up"..."Okay, I think we are getting close now."

With each new message, my heart felt fuller and fuller. I guess the cell service was a little shoddy in there. He had been texting me all along. I still had my Vince, and now it was time for me to support him. He needed his Brett.

Everyone made conversation to pass the time, and I couldn't help thinking how trivial some of the things that they were venting about sounded. *(As if the fact that they had children and a family didn't give them the right to bitch about anything.)* Their lives all seemed so settled. They were so lucky, and they didn't even realize it. After only an hour we got a text that she was already pushing. She had progressed so quickly. We were all shocked. The birth was only a matter of time now. And then all communication went dead silent. We waited. What was once a loud, excited room became quiet and tense.

An hour later all our phones lit up at once. "Baby and Mommy are perfect. Be out soon!"

We all cheered and hugged. Tears of joy. We didn't know the details, but we knew Grace and the baby were safe, and that was a huge relief. All that was left for me was to see Vince. I needed to see his face, to know that he was all right. I needed to know that he still needed me.

We waited for what seemed like hours. Jack had raced back from the city and ran through the door in his suit. He looked so handsome. I still hadn't told him about the two eggs. This was not the time for bad news.

The next time the door opened, it was Vince. "It's a girl!" he shouted.

Everyone waited in line to hug him. When it was my turn, I hoped for something special, but he had too many people to greet.

He was overwhelmed. Happier than I had ever seen him. He looked at peace—more so than I could ever remember. He kept saying how perfect everything went. Her labor was short. She pushed quickly. The baby was perfect. The timing was perfect. All I kept hearing was the word "perfect." It shot through me like a bullet over and over again. Not because I didn't want it to go perfectly for them, but maybe I didn't need to be reminded of how far from perfect I was.

Little by little we were called into the room in small groups to see the baby. Her parents were called in first, and then our family took our turn. As we walked in, I saw Grace with a pink blanket in her arms. My heart melted. Her name was May, and she was beautiful. I wanted to cry. I thought I'd cry. But I didn't. As I walked toward her, Vince followed behind me. He grabbed me, and we held each other. It was longer than a normal hug. He hadn't forgotten. The baby had only made him remember more.

We opened champagne and toasted. I pretended to take a sip since I was in cycle and couldn't drink. I smiled, and I cheered.

But I was pushing away feelings of sorrow for myself. It was so selfish, and I was bitter at God knows who for taking the simple enjoyment out of this for me. It felt like I was wearing a mask of myself.

After the hospital, all I wanted to do was go home. We had to be home for our 7 p.m. shot anyway. Everyone was going to grab something to eat. I tried to say we had to get home, but typical of our family, they convinced us to go. "Come on! Come for one drink."

Jack was on a high from the day and wanted to go. My parents were on cloud nine. My cousins had come. It was time to party.

We sat down at a huge table in the back of a bustling restaurant. I watched the buzzing table as if I was watching a movie of someone else's life. I was numb. An outsider looking in. The room started closing in on me. From under the table, I felt someone grab my hand. It was my mother. She didn't even look at me, nor I at her. She just held my hand tight. In that one moment, I didn't feel so invisible.

I whispered to Jack that I needed to go. I felt an overwhelming sadness crashing in on me, and I was about to lose it. We excused ourselves and walked out.

We barely made it out the door and onto the sidewalk before I burst into tears. He grabbed me and held me tight. He kept saying, "I know. I know." I cried like a baby in his arms. All the pain of the day finally released, all at once, on that very block of cement. I will never forget it.

We drove home just in time for my shot. Jack asked how the doctor visit went. I lied. "Same. Looking good. I'll know more at the next visit." The words just flew out of my mouth. I don't know why I didn't tell him the truth. Maybe I didn't want him to give up hope. Maybe I didn't want him to be disappointed. Or maybe I just wanted to be perfect.

⟡ CHAPTER 28 ⟡

TERROR

There was a terrorist attack today in Battery Park City, on the very street that I used to walk down every single day—the exact path on which my husband used to ride his bike home from work. Should I feel lucky that I wasn't there? Should I feel unlucky that I could've been there? Should it make me forget that I can't have a baby? I know people want me to use it as an excuse to put everything into perspective. But the terror that happened on that street that day doesn't change the terror I feel inside. It doesn't change the fact that I am a shell of myself. And it certainly doesn't change the fact that I have my retrieval tomorrow. What if I don't want perspective? What if I just want a goddamned baby?

The retrieval was scheduled for first thing in the morning. We did the normal routine. We woke up early. Jack showered as I got dressed in cozy pajama pants and a warm baggy sweatshirt. Our interactions always felt forced on these mornings—an odd compilation of awkward movements and trivial conversation as if we were complete strangers interacting on an elevator. Jack sucked down breakfast in the corner of the kitchen, careful not to rub it in that he could eat. I wasn't allowed to have any food or drink for eight hours prior to the retrieval. I couldn't wear jewelry, makeup, or perfumes either. The eggs are very sensitive to any type of scent, so much so that I bought unscented soap to use on the night before my retrievals.

We had all these very strict rules down pat by now, yet my stomach was turning this particular morning, mimicking my thoughts as the various potential outcomes replayed over and over again in my mind. I made a last stop at the bathroom, hoping to avoid farting in the car on the way. You can't blame someone else when there are only two of you in the car. *Side note: I've never farted in front of my husband. Is that weird? Do you?*

As I finished in the bathroom, I turned on the faucet and started to wash my hands. Just as I let out a sigh of relief, I started to smell the intense perfume of the Jo Malone soap I was squirting on my hands. It was a gift from our neighbor when we moved in. The scent was so intense that I had stuck it in a bathroom we rarely used. I stood there reminiscing about how much I hated the smell as I lathered it all over my hands—and then something clicked in my head. The PERFUME RULE! No fragrances! I had completely forgotten.

I screamed, "Jack, Jack!"

"What? What happened?"

"The perfume rule! The soap. The soap!"

"What are you talking about?"

"I used the soap. No fragrances, remember?"

"Oh god, Brett. Well, now what?"

"I don't know. Stop looking at me like that. It was an honest mistake."

"I'm not looking at you. Just trying to figure out what to do."

"By making me feel bad about it?"

This was the last round. What if we had eggs and they died off because of Pomegranate-Lime? Could that happen? I panicked. I ran to the kitchen and saturated my hands in dish soap. "Oh fuck! I did it again!! What am I doing?"

Was this self-sabotage? Had I completely lost my mind? My heart sank, and I began to panic.

Jack started Googling home remedies for removing fragrances from hands. "Okay, here...do we have vinegar and baking soda? You can mix that, and it should do the trick."

I grabbed the ingredients and lathered them all over my hands. I washed them under the water for what seemed like an hour. "I think they smell better. What do you think?"

"I still smell it, but it's definitely lighter," he said. "We really have to go, Brett."

"Okay, Jack, give me a hot second."

I did one more round of washing. When we got in the car, that stupid soap was all I could smell. I tried to sit on my hands to not feed Jack's frustration. *I could've farted in the car after all.*

When we got to RMA, Jack and I were barely speaking. There was so much to say, that we couldn't think of a thing to say. As I was about to walk in the front door, Jack pulled me back and tucked me in close to him. We held each other tight as the frigid morning air gathered around us. I wanted to cry, but I couldn't. I wanted to say something inspirational, but I couldn't. So, I just held on, as if to bask in the glow of not knowing. Out here, I could still hope. Once the doors opened, it was out of our hands.

Jack grabbed my face. "No matter what happens, we have each other. Nothing can change that."

"Not even Jo Malone soap?"

"Especially not Jo Malone soap. Ivory maybe, but definitely not Jo Malone." He looked me deep in the eyes. "I love you, sweetness. Let's do this."

I woke up to the sounds of nurses scurrying around. It took me a few seconds to gather myself and realize where I was. The retrieval was over, and I was alone. All I could see was the blue of the curtains that created walls for my makeshift room. As my blurred vision came into focus, so did the starkness of the situation. I needed to know what happened. It felt like the calm before the storm.

I heard the sound of the curtain swiping against its metal rod as the doctor pushed it to the side. She sat down next to me and held my arm. My body tensed up. She looked me in the eye and smiled. "We were able to retrieve five eggs."

I couldn't believe it. My cheek fell onto the pillow, and I cried. I had never had so many eggs. Was I in a dream? Could this be real? I must have finally got those sleepers I was promised after all! Joy and hope swarmed my heart.

Jack walked into the room. Before he could step all the way past the curtain, I exclaimed, "We have five eggs!" He looked toward the doctor, making sure I wasn't still loopy. She confirmed what I said. He leaned over and hugged me. He was smiling from ear to ear—a smile that I had missed seeing for so long.

The doctor left the room, and Jack followed her out. I knew they were discussing something. When he came back in, he sat down and said nothing. He had a weird look on his face.

"You aren't seriously thinking about not telling me what you were just talking to the doctor about, are you?"

"It's not a big deal but, well, when I went in to 'do my thing' I sort of missed...the cup."

"Um, run that by me again?"

"I missed the cup. I mean not completely but enough."

I let out a calm "Okay, okay," but on the inside I was going ape shit. My trusty partner in all this! So, his "perfect sperm" missed their ride to the game? How does that happen? Doesn't matter now that they are perfect, does it, Cheng? Doesn't matter now!

He mumbled, "Enough got in though, I think."

"Oh, okay, well as long as you think enough got in."

Don't worry about it. After all, I only had four rounds of needles in my stomach, hot flashes, bloating, not drinking, not exercising, not shitting, sleeping, or socializing, as I crop-dusted everyone in my life with my shit ass moods for the past year. But as long as you "think" it all got in.

Still, the look of horror on his face made my heart melt. We were in this together. I reached over and grabbed his hand. "Maybe the pomegranate-lime will wake up the ones that did get in the cup."

He laughed and smirked at me, knowing full well I was letting him off the hook. We officially had all our eggs in one basket. It was both exciting and terrifying at the same time.

The waiting for the results was always so harsh, harsher than any physical symptom during the rounds. The waiting was cruel. We were so helpless. Everything else took a backseat during these times. Work, seeing friends, even talking to each other. We would watch the hours pass, willing them to go by faster. I didn't know how to feel, but with five eggs retrieved, we had some numbers to work with. The number of viable eggs always dwindled. When you start with two, zero wasn't far behind. But five was different! We had a real shot here. When the doctor called and said only three of the five had fertilized, I knew we were still in the ring, fighting to survive. Fighting to not be counted out.

We had five more days to wait to see if these matured. I became sick to my stomach. My high from the retrieval had barely worn off when the usual feelings of hopelessness unfairly tried to drag me back into the hole. But I wouldn't let that happen this time. This would work.

Five morning showers, where I stood lifeless, fixated on the water striking the back of my neck, then pummeling to my feet. Five wasted workdays where nothing seemed important. Five days of calls sent to voicemail, as I couldn't bear to hear the pep talks of my family and friends. For five days, time stood still as I crawled closer to the crossroad that would either way change my life forever.

The doctor called on day five like clockwork, exposing the exact science of it all. Two eggs had survived the maturing stage and could be sent for genetic testing. Was I thrilled? Was I disappointed? Was I petrified? Was I hopeful? Was I starting to remember the familiar feelings of rounds before? Yes. All of the above. We had two weeks of more waiting for the genetic testing results—the last stage in our waiting game. Though we were close, though we were still in the game, and though there was nothing more we could do, the anticipation was breaking me.

↗ CHAPTER 29 ↖

FEELING RED

Do you know that girl among your husband's friends that for whatever reason you just get a funny feeling around? The one who makes you feel like she's going to steal your husband the second you don't show up to a party? I'm not a jealous type. Jack has plenty of female friends, and I have no issues with them. It's just this one. She's blonde and has some high-powered job on Wall Street. She's the girl who shows up to a party in a baseball hat and looks sexier than you in the dolled-up outfit you spent all day preparing. The one who somehow gets her nipples to show perfectly through her shirt without it looking tacky. The girl who goes out of her way to subtly remind you that you aren't part of their past. Well, we have one of those. Her name is Sierra. And for all of these reasons I spent weeks dreading seeing her at this engagement party we had coming up.

As the weekend came closer, I felt more and more anxious. I had nothing to wear, I felt swollen, my hormones were exploding, and I had nothing to show for my life since I had seen this gang at our wedding two years before. They all knew about the IVF, and we had no news to share. It all added up to a recipe for disaster—a *perfect storm* that would attack my life about ten minutes before we had to leave when I still had nothing to wear.

Seeing her was all I could think about. I followed her on Facebook, where I could see that she was living the life. In the Hamptons one weekend, Iceland the next. Relaxing on boats with cool people. Posting lyrics of old rock songs. She had this tight curly hair that always looked messy in the most glorious way possible. The type of hair that I have spent hundreds of dollars in salt sprays trying to master. Her cool factor was irritating.

It was Thursday, and the party was Friday, in New York, where she lived. Where I no longer did. Not sure how I let this slip out of my grasp, but with only twenty-four hours to go, I had nothing to wear, needed to lose ten pounds, and somehow had to find my mojo. One glance at her with her young, sprite ovaries was sure to push me over the edge. I felt like I had lost even before we arrived.

I woke up that morning and got ready for work like I always did. As I walked out to my car, I saw a note waiting there. It was from Jack. *Can't wait to spend the weekend with you, beauty.* What was I doing?

It wasn't like me to give up. I realized that I had to fight. Fight for myself. Fight for my dignity. Fight for my goddamn husband! I had to find the person who I knew was still somewhere deep inside me.

I was determined to show up to the party looking as good as I possibly could—to feel good about myself again and be proud of who I was. I started my car and started to drive. I passed the exit for work. There was no time to waste on work. I passed the exit for the Short Hills Mall. This job was bigger than the mall. There was only one way to fix this. INTERMIX. I turned the radio up, put my foot on the gas, and headed toward the Holland Tunnel. This Tribeca girl was coming home.

There's always that moment while shopping overweight when you have to come to grips with the fact that you need to get the larger size. It usually takes a few pulls gone wrong. You have to swallow your pride, get dressed again, and walk back out to the floor to start from scratch. The problem is, in INTERMIX, bigger sizes are essentially nonexistent, and when you ask for them, especially at five-foot-two, they death-stare you down. As if to say, *Really? Get your shit together.* I kind of like that about the place. I tried on dress after dress. Nothing was zipping, let alone looking good. The dressing room was a graveyard of outfits that could have been—like ghosts of Christmas past. Just before I was about to have a complete mental breakdown, Stella McCartney saved my life. The dress was the boldest red I had ever seen. It was too short. It was too tight. It was perfect. Did it look like I needed a bigger size? Yes. Did it completely show my IVF gut? Absolutely. But when I looked in that mirror, I felt sexy as hell. I stared at myself. Is that really me? The appeal went beyond the dress, though, and beyond the fact that my ass looked amazing in it.

It struck something within me. I saw my old self. I saw the confidence, the strength. The swagger of the girl I used to be. I was a woman. A woman who was going through IVF. A woman I wanted to be.

Next stop, The Dry Bar. If this girl was going down, she was going down swinging—with a head full of perfectly blow-dried hair.

It was a beautiful autumn night. The city felt alive, and I was on fire. For the first time in almost a year, I felt amazing. Sierra had no chance. Not tonight. Tonight belonged to me. She would look me up and down and panic. That's right, from the slate shimmer on my eyes down to the gold Louboutins on my feet, and I was going to enjoy every second of it. Little did she know I would be sucking in so hard I would barely be able to breathe. But hey, priorities. Jack greeted me with a "LOOK at you!" His eyes lit up. I knew immediately that I had her beat.

We walked into the cocktail hour, and I started to look for her. She was nowhere to be found. Knowing that she was probably watching somewhere, I made sure to nestle closer to Jack. Securing the piss on my territory. We made our way into the ballroom. There she was, sitting in a corner. She was in flats and a black dress. Her hair looked dull, and she had a weird look on her face. As she got up to greet us, I saw it. A plastic tube taped to her arm. My heart sank. Dragging behind her was an IV.

I didn't know why she had it, but it didn't matter. In that moment I wanted to rip that dress off my body so fast. I felt ashamed. All I wanted to do was look worse than she did. I wanted her to win. When she looked up at me, I could see the humiliation on her face. Who had I become? I wanted to say that I was sorry. Sorry that she had to go through whatever it was she was going through. Sorry that she must have dreaded coming to this party for weeks. Sorry that she probably had no idea what to wear. And sorry that she was feeling anything but the greatest version of herself.

The IVF process opens your heart for anyone else who is going through something. Whatever it is. Just anything that makes you feel like a piece of yourself is gone. I saw myself in her hopelessness. I wanted to comfort her, but it wasn't my place. I wanted to connect with her, but I didn't know how. I felt like an asshole. I pushed out my gut as far as it would go, walked toward her, and hugged her. I hugged her as long and as hard as I could. I whispered in her ear, "You've got this."

She pulled back, looked me deep into the eyes, and said, "So do you."

♪ CHAPTER 30 ♩

A SHITSTORM

Someone shit on our floor today. Yes, you heard that right. One of our workers got mad at a manager and actually took a giant dump in the middle of the plant floor and walked out. So, while all you distinguished young executives were ringing the Wall Street bell and coming up with the next big marketing campaign, I was figuring out how to deal with what the repercussions would be for someone defecating in the workplace. In all fairness, Vince was the one who actually had to deal with it. I just got to be completely and utterly entertained by it and make fun of him from behind the scenes. So you can only imagine how hysterical it was for me when he had to bring the entire company together to have a "meeting" about pooping on floors, as if now there was a new company policy and shitting on the floor would no longer be allowed. It was glorious.

When the meeting started, I stood way in the back, trying my hardest not to make eye contact with Vince. I didn't want to set off one of those "can't laugh in class" moments. My knowing he had to take it so seriously and his knowing that I was taking it so not seriously was the perfect recipe for disaster. The funniest part was that after he spoke a few sentences, a translator had to repeat what he said in Spanish for our Spanish-speaking employees. For some reason, that made the whole thing even funnier.

Given such dire circumstances, I knew there was only one thing to do—video it. I slowly reached into my purse and grabbed my phone. I kept it close to my side, making sure that no one saw me. As I glanced down to switch my phone to video mode, I saw a voice message—from RMA. This could only mean the results were in.

My head jerked up, and I stared straight ahead. Suddenly, the room felt empty and any humor I found was sucked away. I stood there cold. Voices became muffled as my thoughts echoed within the walls of my head. My phone felt heavy. It carried my fate. I ran through every scenario in my mind. All I wanted was one embryo. Just one. Two would be amazing. Just any outcome other than none.

I slowly bowed my way out of the meeting, catching Vince's eye as I walked toward my office. I shut my door behind me and sat down. I could feel beads of sweat forming on my neck as my stomach twisted into knots. I slowly brought the phone to my ear and pressed voicemail. Waiting for it to come on was the longest few seconds of my life. I heard Nurse Adrienne's voice as she started to speak.

The door opened to my office, and Vince came in, laughing about what had just happened. Surprised when he didn't see me joking back, he shut the door behind him. I lost all control of my emotions.

"It worked, Vince. It worked."

I cried harder as I went on, in between hiccups. "They are both good. They are both good! We have two embryos!"

He came close and hugged me. I cried hysterically in his arms. I had finally been thrown a lifeline after treading water for a year. He held me tight. He kissed the top of my head. He stayed calm, hesitant to claim this as a victory just yet. He knew I still had a long way to go.

I had to tell Jack—in person. He was working from home that day, and I didn't know if I could last for the thirty-minute car ride it would take to get to him. I had to tell him face to face. I got my coat and ran toward the exit. As I turned the corner toward the parking lot...there he was...standing there. Jack had beaten me to the punch. The doctor had called him after they couldn't get in touch with me.

I ran into his arms. We held each other. Our embrace felt different than ever before. For the first time ever, I saw him cry. Though there were still hurdles to overcome, this nightmare might actually become a dream come true after all.

We had two viable embryos! We. Had. Two. Embryos.

CHAPTER 31

CECILIA, YOU'RE BREAKING MY HEART

Logically, the first question that everyone asked me was: when was I going to put the embryos back in? Seems like a simple enough question. But the process was more complicated than that. Though we had two, that did not mean that we would have two children necessarily. Dr. Scott told us that you really need two embryos for every one pregnancy. In other words, there was no guarantee that either embryo would take.

This bit of information freaked me out. I labored over the decision of whether or not to put those two embryos on hold and go for a fifth round of retrieval or go straight to the transfer of one of them. On the one hand, maybe I was on a roll and I shouldn't quit trying to find eggs while I was younger. I was so delayed at this point. On the other hand, though, if I was going to commit to having another round, I would have to commit to multiple rounds. That made the point even harder to swallow. The thought of going through it again made me feel sick. But I wanted to look back and say that I did everything I could do for our family. Just because we had problems getting to this point didn't mean I had to let go of my vision of having multiple children someday. Was that greedy? Was I not allowed to have that dream anymore? After this last round was a success, I knew that the next would be too. I just knew it.

Everyone thought I was crazy for even thinking about doing more rounds. (My father even asked me if I was addicted to IVF.) Part of me felt the desire was a bit insane. But the thought was logical, no? Didn't anyone get it? It wasn't just about having the one child. It was about completing my vision.

Everyone responded differently. One common response was, "Why don't you just put in both and have twins?" That made me angry. As if it were all so easy. The doctors don't just do that. And what if they did? Why would I be so wasteful with my embryos, anyway? Why wouldn't I want two tries? I've never been pregnant before. What if I had trouble holding a pregnancy? In the back of my mind lingered a fear that our journey may be far from over. And that haunted me.

Jack left the decision up to me. He said at this point it was my body, and I had been through so much already. When the doctor called, asking for my final decision regarding whether to move forward with a fifth round, I still hadn't made up my mind. In a moment of crazy optimism, I said, "Let's do it." I dragged myself back into the game. Round Five was officially underway.

Three weeks and one day later, I opened my eyes to the same

curtains around me that I had seen four times before. All I could hear was the sound of muffled voices and nurses moving in the hall. The fifth retrieval was over. As I reached consciousness, a wave of agony tore through my abdomen. I had never felt anything like that with the other four retrievals. Did something go wrong? It felt like stabbing waves of pressure shooting through my uterus every few minutes. I was alone and in too much pain to call out. In my delirium, all I could think about was the retrieval and how many eggs they were able to pull. I was obsessed—like a drug addict in withdrawal. My body was clearly telling me I had gone too far.

The next thing I remember was Jack lying on the bed beside me. He couldn't make eye contact with me. He just held me close. "No eggs survived the retrieval this time, babe. I'm so sorry."

The physical pain was now overtaken by the mental anguish. We were back to where we had started a month before. The entire round was a waste. A devastating waste.

I turned toward the wall. I couldn't bear to see the look on his face, knowing he wanted me to stop, knowing I had to keep going.

"We need to seriously think about what we want to do moving forward. It's hard, Brett. It's hard."

"I know it's hard, Jack. You don't think I know it's hard?" I asked.

"I mean, it's hard for me to see you like this. This isn't what I want for you."

I lay there, realizing the harsh reality that I was alone in my insanity. I was hurting those closest to me, even though I knew in my heart that there had to be more eggs.

When the doctor came back in, I heard her say, "swollen uterus," "kinking," and "spasms." I wasn't even listening. All I could think about was my next move. Did I have a sixth retrieval in me? I had to keep going, *right*? As I lay there for a few hours, the physical pain became better, but the conflict in my mind became worse. I was tired and frustrated—like I had run a marathon in place. I was more conflicted than ever. My body was clearly telling me to stop, but my heart was telling me to keep going. I felt more alone than ever in my decision to want to try for a sixth round. Irrationality was taking over.

One week later, I had to take a client to dinner in New York. My client, who was already three sheets to the wind, left to catch his train. I was alone as I finished paying the bill. The remnants of random appetizers littered the table as I sat there circling the top of my half-drunken wine glass with my finger. I had to summon the energy for my commute home. I finally grabbed my jacket and headed toward the exit.

As I was walking out, I looked toward the bar and saw a familiar face out of the corner of my eye. A girl I went to college with. She was a few years older than I. I didn't know her well, but I recognized her face. She had blond hair, soft blue eyes, and a pale pretty complexion that hadn't changed since college. I don't know what made me turn back around, but I did. Once we locked eyes, I had no choice but to make my way toward her.

"You went to Bucknell, right? Janine? I'm Brett Russo. Not sure if you remember me or not."

"Yes, I do. You married Jack, right?"

"I did. So funny. What brings you here?"

"I work right around the corner. I missed my train, so I figured I'd have a drink while I waited for the next one."

"I just finished a client dinner. About to jump on a train myself."

Trying to continue the small talk, she asked, "So where are you living now?"

"Well, we moved to New Jersey in July. Really loving it but definitely missing the city."

Then came the ever-present unavoidable question. "Do you have any children?"

Trying to squeeze out a smile, I answered, "Not yet. You?"

"Yes, we actually have a little girl. Her name is Cecilia. She's three. She has definitely changed our lives."

"I'm sure. That's what I hear. Well, Cecilia is a beautiful name." I felt myself pulling away, ready to make my exit, but something held me in place. The look on her face. I couldn't quite put my finger on it. Without thinking, I heard myself say the words that I was so quick to hide from most people. "We've been having some trouble having a baby. Going through IVF actually."

Her eyes teared up immediately as she reached for my hand. "I'm so sorry you had to go through that."

"You don't have to be sorry—"

She grabbed my hand harder as she interrupted, "No, Brett, I'm truly sorry you have to go through this. We went through six rounds ourselves before Cecilia. It honestly almost broke me."

With that, I signaled to the bartender. "We're going to need a bottle of your best Pinot Noir. And by best, I mean the cheapest one on the menu."

She laughed and then started to open up to me about everything that happened to her. Her battle. Her miscarriages. Her mental struggles. Before I knew it, we were three glasses deep, and I was glued to her every word. Her bravery in opening up to me, essentially a stranger, about the hardest time in her life, was something I will never forget. Someone was finally speaking my language. After everything she went through, she came out on top. As she talked, I thought to myself how she was one of the lucky ones. She came out on the other side with a child. I wanted to be a lucky one too.

She spoke about her daughter with such amazement and love. I'd never experienced anything like it. "Would you like to see a picture of her?"

"I'd love to."

She pulled out her phone and swiped around. She then handed it to me. "This was the first time I held her." I looked down at the picture and saw her holding a beautiful brown-skinned baby girl. I looked up, caught off-guard at seeing Cecilia's dark skin. "She was only a month old when we got her."

I looked back down at the photo. I couldn't peel my eyes away. I will never forget the look of love in Janine's eyes in that picture. It was that of a woman who had fought the battle of her life and won. But it was the look on the baby's face that struck me more. This helpless, beautiful little girl needing a mother's love so desperately. There was something about it that I couldn't shake.

It dawned on me then that this journey was not about my egg count, my retrievals, or the countless injections. It was about being a mother—no matter what my path was to get there. Seeing Janine's baby look up at her mom with her helpless eyes and Janine looking back with a look of unspoken love telling her adopted daughter, "You are home," awakened a deep yearning inside me. Seeing them together made me realize that my dreams were closer than I thought. No matter what the details were. It was that simple after all. I had gotten so far removed from what this all actually meant. The road forward was suddenly crystal clear.

I gave Janine a long, hard hug and thanked her. She took the cork from our bottle of wine off the bar and put it in my hand. She hugged me one more time before she ran off to the train. "You'll get through this too. Put that embryo in. And always know that if it doesn't work, you can still be a mother. Don't be afraid to change your ending."

I sat there staring at the cork in my hand, finding all the answers I ever needed. Being a mother was so much more than the origin of an egg or sperm. Seeing that picture made the mere concept of it seem trivial even. It was about unconditional love. It was about holding the only baby you were ever meant to have in your arms.

Janine probably had no idea what she had done for me that night. I went outside and dialed Jack's number. When he picked up the phone, I uttered the words that I never thought I would say:

"No matter how I get there, I'm ready to be a mother."

⟋ CHAPTER 32 ⟍

A NEW YEAR

Nothing says the holidays like two embryos and a transfer on the way. Sounds like a Christmas carol: *"Five rounds of grief! Four mental breakdowns, three lost friends, two embryos, and a year of not waxing my bush."* Magical. It was December, and we decided to take a month off to let my body have a break. Our transfer was scheduled for January 23. Hope was swirling in the air, and we were ready to enjoy the time away from IVF. After seeing Janine, all I could think about was being a mom, yet I was uncomfortable getting too far ahead of myself. Maybe I was scarred by the last year, like a battered puppy that flinches when you try to pet it. I tried not to wrap my head around too many scenarios. If I've learned anything in this process, it's don't write your ending before it happens. All I knew was, I could breathe again. I actually caught my husband flirting with me again. We even had sex. *Just kidding.* Let's not get crazy. Who has sex anymore?

New Year's Eve! The night when everyone gets dressed up in their finest clothes and pops champagne bottles while they go out to fancy dinners and parties—unless you're a wife of a Phish fan. And then, well, you go to Madison Square Garden to hear them play jam band music and bobble your head for four hours while ex-hippies sweat all over you as you listen to jams that last forty-five minutes long. So that's what we did. We were in such a good place that I had to be beside Jack when the clock struck midnight.

The night took on a life of its own. We had started at some dive bar and got a great buzz on. I hadn't been drunk in a year, and honestly, it felt amazing. We had met up with a few friends of ours who were going as well. Just when I felt like the night couldn't get any better, in walked Tom. You know Tom. Our good friend from high school? The one married to Camila from the BBQ who froze her eggs, called it IVF, and sent me home in tears? Yeah, that Tom. Seeing him was the icing on the cake. We had a crew, we had a vibe, and we had a buzz. It was a recipe for the greatest New Year's Eve ever.

The first set went off, and for the first time, I actually got lost in the music. Jack and I danced and swayed as they played songs that we recognized. It was the happiest I could remember being in so long. A night we needed so badly. A night we deserved. When the lights came back on, we all sat in our seats, excited for the next set to start. Jack went to get us drinks, and Tom and I sat there catching up. "So, I have something to tell you," he said. Caught off-guard by his sly tone, I was intrigued to hear what was coming next. He looked at me, smiled, and said, "Camila's pregnant."

I looked at him. Okay, okay. You know what? I could handle this. We had our two embryos, and I was going to be ok. Though it was hard to hear about yet another person having a baby, I owed him my happiness, and I wanted to give it to him. I took a breath, dug deep, and hugged him.

"It happened on the first try. I can't believe how easy it was!" He kept going on and on about that particular aspect of it. And for whatever reason, that was the straw that broke the camel's back. By the time Jack came back with the drinks, I was running toward the bathroom.

I went to the farthest stall, shut the door, and started to cry. I realized how close I still was to those feelings of despair. Just when I thought I had them beat, they resurfaced, reminding me how immersed in this I still was. Why tonight? Why her? Did a part of me hope that someday she would understand how she made me feel? *Maybe.* Did alcohol play a role? *Probably.* Did everyone else in my life respect me enough to tell us in private with enough time to soak it in and respond? *Definitely.* But all those factors, combined with the reality of our still precarious position, buried me alive, and I couldn't pull myself together.

As the music came back on, I knew it was only a matter of time before Jack would start to worry about me. I didn't want to ruin his night or anyone else's. I didn't know what to do. I was hoping some Birkenstock-wearing hippie chick would come to my rescue, but she probably took one look at my INTERMIX platform heels from below the stall and kept walking. Eventually, I heard Jack calling my name from the doorway. I washed my face and walked out. I couldn't hide the fact that I had been crying. We got our stuff and walked out of the concert without saying goodbye. The night was lost, and it was all my fault.

As we got in the cab, I apologized. Jack merely smiled and pulled me closer to him as I laid my head on his shoulder. As the cab approached the tunnel, we heard the cheers from the streets. It was midnight. We sat there in silence holding each other. Numb. Inside our own thoughts, present only in touch. The year was finally over. And a new fight had just begun.

CHAPTER 33

TAKE A CHANCE ON ME

The transfer prep was under way! What the hell is a transfer anyway? Well, I'm going to tell you. Our little embryo had been frozen for two months now. When the timing was right, they would let the embryo thaw and put it back inside my uterus. Then we would wait ten days to see if it implanted in the lining of the uterus. If it did, I was pregnant. If it didn't then, well, I wasn't. It's that simple.

The prep was much easier than the prep for the retrieval. It consisted of readying my body to be pregnant, which really meant staying as healthy as possible. In order to get the lining of the uterus thick enough for the embryo to implant you take a pill called estradiol for fifteen days before the transfer. About five days before the transfer, I began to get progesterone shots, which are injections into the muscle, also known as a big ass needle in your butt. When you're pregnant, your body naturally produces progesterone so that the uterus can grow. These injections supplement the progesterone that the body would make if you got pregnant naturally. It gives the body what it needs until it can kick in and start producing enough on its own. Those shots would continue for eight weeks into my pregnancy. Okay. Class dismissed.

The world felt alive. I was inspired by the idea that my dream was on the brink of coming true. I felt like I had already won. We had come so far. On the other hand, I was nervous about what this next stage would bring. We had jumped the first hurdle, which was producing viable embryos. But what if that was only the start? What if I couldn't maintain a pregnancy? What if I miscarried? What if the journey was far from over? It was hard not to think of all the negative possibilities; my brain had become trained to think that way as a defense mechanism.

I still had, though, the certainty that I would be a mother no matter what. It radiated through me like a comet, bouncing off the inside walls of my body over and over again. I was still too close to the journey, afraid to look back, as if it would suck me back in. I had no choice but to look forward.

Everyone kept telling me that this is where my good health would kick in and play a positive role. But what if it didn't work? Would it then be my fault? All I had left was my dream; the vision of my children someday hiding behind the curtains in my dining room. The vision of my little one playing with cousins under the table and next to the Christmas tree. I dug hard and deep. I knew I had more fight inside of me. I wasn't empty yet. It was time to get back in touch with my inner soldier—the woman who my mother taught me to be and the positive girl who came before her. It was our turn to finish the story that I would tell my grandchildren someday. It was our turn to have the only thing we ever wanted: a chance.

On the morning of the transfer, I was lying wide awake in my bed well before dawn. I didn't sleep that night, and by the time 5 a.m. rolled around, I knew any chance of sleep was gone. I walked around my room, pacing from one end to the other, wondering what the day would bring. I watched Jack as he slept. He was still wearing headphones and an iPad lay next to his head—his tools to help him fight the urge to think last night. As I walked toward the closet, I ran my fingers along the top of the dresser that I had stared at for so many sleepless nights, month after month, wondering what would happen to me. Missing a child I never had. Wishing for a life that was slipping from my grasp.

I walked into the closet, where the bag I had started to pack for the day lay open. I grabbed some socks and some loosely fitting underwear from the drawer and added them. My eyes grazed past a pile I had been keeping of all the things that people had been giving me throughout this process. I had saved every single note, bead, and relic. They gave me strength. Though each one addressed a different stage in my journey, their message was the same: don't give up, I am right beside you.

I reached for a fertility crystal that Grace had given me, and I held it in my hand. A friend of hers who went through IVF gave it to her so she could give to me. I remembered so clearly when she did. I remember thinking that a woman in my shoes held this same crystal in her hands during her darkest moments. It held her tears and her triumphs. But most of all, it held her prayers. I found comfort in that. I couldn't leave it behind. I gave it one last glance, turned around, and placed it in my bag.

Behind that I saw the necklace that Jaci had given me during my first IVF cycle. The light gold chain held a tiny bird charm. I wore it around my neck during that entire first round. It was with me from the very start. That seemed so long ago. I held it close to my chest, remembering the hardships and shock of those first few results. I turned around and placed it next to the crystal.

As I sifted through the pile, these mementos recalled every story of my journey. From the notes, copper pennies, socks, bracelets, fertility beads, prayer cards, right down to the cork that Janine gave me just a few weeks ago, I realized that I couldn't leave any of it behind. Like a childhood teddy bear, they held all my hopes, dreams, and all of the tears I hid from the world. Before I knew it the pile of all those things that once sat on my dresser was gathered in my bag. There was no better place for them than by my side today. I needed them more than ever.

I got dressed and walked out to the kitchen. The morning spoke to me as it had so many times before. I wrapped myself in a big blanket and walked out onto our porch. The air was cold and crisp. It felt fresh and new. I sat down on the stone steps. The cold stung my bottom through the blanket. I watched the sun rise through the shadows that crept across the lawn. The silent morning air played music. My thoughts were clear. The day was here, and there was nothing left to fear.

By the time Jack woke up, I was back in the kitchen with music playing and egg whites and turkey bacon sizzling on the stovetop.

"Let's go, Daddy, time for breakfast," I said as I tried to maneuver the pan in the air to flip the bacon cooking on top.

Though I'm sure it wasn't what he expected, he played along like a champ. "Well, look at the master chef. How long were you working on that?"

"First time," I sarcastically responded, pretending to ignore the fact that the bacon had missed the pan and gone all over the floor.

He came up behind me and hugged me, bringing his face to the back of my neck. I could feel him breathing. We both knew what was at stake, and nothing was going to distract us from that no matter what we did. JAY-Z tried as he sang songs from our college days through the Sonos speaker. "If you're having girl problems, I feel bad for you, son," Jack lip-synched as he waved his hands up and down in the air.

"Drop the mic and come sit down and eat. This could be the last time we are only two."

"Well, you better work on your bacon-flipping skills, then."

Though we joked, the charged air between us was exciting and terrifying all at the same time. It was safe to say that like the song, "We had 99 problems...but a bitch wasn't one."

When we arrived at RMA, Jack turned off the car. My hand was on the door, but I wasn't quite ready to open it yet.

"You ready for this, kid?"

I took a long breath in. "Does a pope shit in the woods?"

"You mean bear?"

"No, I mean pope."

"Of course you do. Time to do this, sweetness." He got out and walked around the car toward my door.

Left alone, I took my last breath in. I've got this. I've got this. He opened my door and helped me out. We walked in hand in hand.

We were directed to a section we had never been to before. The doors were right by the entrance. I had passed them a hundred times, and I always wondered what went on there. I finally knew. We walked into the room assigned for us and sat down. The nurse came in and sat down next to me. "An Eagles jersey, huh? You don't see too much of that around here."

"Well, my husband here is from Philly. I told him I'd give him the Eagles, but I was keeping my Yankees."

"Smart call." She continued to talk us through the procedure. We had to sign some papers and then we waited.

The first person that came in was the acupuncturist. Research RMA had conducted showed that acupuncture increases your chances of a successful transfer if done before and after the procedure, so of course we opted to do it. It was called laser acupuncture. The man handed Jack and me huge sunglasses and asked us to put them on. We looked like we had just had couple's cataract surgery. We tried not to laugh, careful not to offend the acupuncturist, who seemed awfully serious and tense for, well, an acupuncturist.

I was given instructions to take three deep breaths and relax my body. With each breath in, I tried to capture all the stress of the year before and then expel it up through my chest and away from my body. I felt like being at peace through this process was important. There was only good ahead. I tried to speak to my own body. Calming myself. Believing in myself. Clearing all the negative karma from my aura. Preparing this baby's new home. It was a deeper moment than I had anticipated. The magnitude of the situation building excitement in my gut. I believed it would work.

The next person who came into the room was Dr. Hong. She was a beautiful young doctor with a warm face that felt soothing to see especially on a day like today. "Nurse Adrienne told me I had to take good care of you. You are one of her favorites." There she was, Nurse Adrienne, fighting in the background for me once again. My Drill Sergeant. My angel. My friend. Who knows if she said that about all her patients? But today, I felt like her favorite, like people were in my corner. Behind her was a nurse, then the embryologist, and behind her...

I gasped, "Jack, it's our embryo."

It was brought in a clear incubator-like case on a cart. I couldn't believe my eyes. It never felt more real than it did right then. My heart stopped. Jack and I both looked at each other and couldn't help but tear up. Everything we had been through had come down to this. He inched his chair close to where I was lying and grabbed my hand. "You okay?"

"I'm goddamned amazing."

The doctor started to get ready. We could see every move on a screen next to the bed. The embryologist wheeled the embryo toward me. "Now, I need you to take a deep breath and relax," the doctor said as she pushed her chair toward the edge of the bed.

It was time. I slowly put my feet up into the stirrups. My legs were trembling. Dr. Hong put her hand on my knee and smiled. "You're ready for this."

I nodded and laid back.

She signaled to the nurse, as her warm sweet face changed to intensely focused, like someone had changed the human being inside. She was not here to mess around. In that moment, it became clear how seriously she took this job.

The embryologist picked up the embryo with a special syringe and carefully handed it to Dr. Hong. I watched on the screen as she placed the tool inside me.

"Okay, you will see my syringe go in. There we go," she spoke slowly as she concentrated. "See it there? I'm releasing it now. See all that fluid? Your embryo is in there."

The sensation was unbelievable. I tried to stay relaxed and stay at peace. Despite all the people in the room, all I could feel was me and that embryo—as if everyone else had melted away. *Stay strong, my little one. You and me. We've got this. You have to stay strong a little longer.*

I held Jack's hand tighter and tighter. Everything in the room went blank except for that screen. I was witnessing for the first time our possible child. Reunited with me. Home. Where it belonged. The doctor slowly removed the syringe, and the screen went blank. Jack and I unlocked our hands, which were clammy with sweat. Just like that, the procedure was over. Little embryo was on its own now.

I lay there not wanting to move a muscle—my body tense and my mind full. Dr. Hong placed her hands on the top of my knees and stared at me as she connected with something inside of me. I reached toward her and grabbed her hand on my knee as I started to cry. She held my hand back just as tight. "You change people's lives. There's no way to thank you." I said as I wiped the tears from my eyes. She stared at me a bit longer as the warmth of her face flooded back. "You just did. Good luck to you." She stared into my eyes a bit longer and then left the room. It's a moment I'll never forget.

The nurse remained and explained how I had to treat my body as if I were pregnant. She went through some rules of what I should and shouldn't do. I had heard all of it before. No alcohol, lunch meats, sushi, etc...She said that walking around this afternoon would help the embryo to implant into the uterine lining, more so than just lying down and resting. I soaked in all she was saying and tried to make sense out of everything that had just happened. Ten minutes ago, it was just Jack and I, and now we could be three.

Watching this all unfold in front of me, I couldn't help but wonder how everyone's prayers played in this process. What was God's role in all of this? What I had gone through felt so scientific. Hadn't I just witnessed a doctor creating life? I looked up and asked, "So what's the next step?"

"Well, you're going to come back in ten days from now for a pregnancy blood test to see if it attached to the uterine lining."

"Okay, and then what?"

"A few weeks after that, you come in for an ultrasound to see if the heart started beating."

"So how do you get the heart to start beating?"

She smiled at me and laughed. "Oh, we can't control that. It either starts beating or it doesn't."

I just looked at her. It all became hauntingly clear. They had figured out a way to retrieve an egg from a mother's body. They found a way to fertilize it with the father's sperm. They even had a way to put it back inside the mother and help it to implant into the uterine lining. But there was one thing that they as doctors couldn't do. There was one thing they hadn't figured out: How to get that heart to start beating. How to give it life.

Was it luck? *Could be.* Was it science? *Partly.* But maybe it was more than that. I closed my eyes, brought my hands together, and did something I hadn't done in years. I prayed.

CHAPTER 34

IT TAKES A VILLAGE

Before I go on, there's a chapter that needs to be written—a chapter about the people that have stood by us. I mean, *really* stood by us. You will be surprised who they end up being. They are my true angels. I have counted on them in ways that I can't begin to describe. The people who gave me strength every day—the weekly calls and texts of inspiration, the check-ins, the cards I got in the mail, and the random gifts of fertility bracelets, crystals, copper pennies, and prayer cards. *I never knew my friends were so religious.* Anyone seeing them on my counter would think I was about to join a nunnery.

There are also those little laughs along the way. Weekly IVF cartoon pics containing turkey basters and talking sperm from one cousin, while the other told me that this was just God's way of preparing me for the misery of being a mother. My father constantly asking me, "Are you sure Jack's doing it right?" It sounds silly and maybe demented, but I counted on these welcome laughs as some of my only relief. These are the people who make me feel whole again. Just when I think I'm going to lose it, I'm reminded of how loved I am.

I've found that it's hard to tell people on the outside what you're going through. Sometimes you open up to someone, thinking they will understand, and they just look at you blankly and say, "It will happen," and then walk away. I'm always jealous of their ability to walk away and put it out of their minds. But one thing I've tried to remember is that you can't blame anyone for not knowing what to say or for shying away because they don't know how to handle something. Even some of your closest friends may not realize how hard this process is, especially since they haven't been through it. Most people know very little about IVF, so you have to focus on the people who are there for you and their positive energy. If they haven't left your side by now, they won't. At least I hope not.

My mother fields a call from me every day, unless there is news to tell and then we're on the phone multiple times a day. She just listens and lets me cry, bitch, or feel bad for myself, and then she attempts to lift me back up. I don't know how she does it. She never seems annoyed or tired of hearing about my struggles. It's almost as if she is going through IVF with us. She has taught me so much about being a mother.

As for my brother, Vince, he has the misfortune of always being with me when I get all the tough news, but he is hurting right along with us. For some reason that makes me feel better, not because I want him to be in pain, but sharing the grief with someone else somehow makes it easier to bear. Vince lets me vent but then doesn't let me feel sorry for myself. He doesn't let me drift down the pity river too long before he says, "That's what it is, Brett. You have to keep going."

Another person by my side is my wacky cousin Jaci. She believes in fate, the universe, beads, and God. She literally keeps a bag of holy statues in her purse. One has a head that fell off, but she keeps it anyway. Whenever we fly anywhere, she lays them all out on the fold-down tray table. People think we're nuts, but we don't care. She sends me chapters of inspirational texts, with random cards and gifts always pleasantly surprising me in the mail.

My cousin Marla, who lives in London, will pick up the phone at any hour of the day to take an upsetting call from me. She's also the cousin who told me to go "fuck" myself on a Happy Mother's Day text stream. It was the perfect dysfunctional reminder I needed to laugh at myself.

Some of the most supportive people are those that have been through it. Sarah is my friend from college. The doctors told her she would never have her own children, and now she wheels around a specially made stroller fit for four. I'll never forget the first time I called her. We hadn't spoken in years. I heard her voice on the other end of the phone and just started to cry. She knew. She didn't need any backstory. After all the rough results, she helped guide me through the process. Martine, who even through ten rounds of IVF and three miscarriages, always took the time out of her own grief to be there for me. Janine, who after six rounds of IVF and countless ups and downs, adopted a beautiful baby girl who she loves fiercely. She opened up to me about every detail, making me feel less alone in my search for answers. Francine, who used an egg donor and who has walked me through the process as many times as I needed. Heather and Steven used a surrogate, and their bravery was a true inspiration for me. Steven checked in on me every single day and at times was more insightful than my doctors. And these are just a few. These women were brave enough to let me in and to share their stories with me. I feel so blessed in this way. These are the people who were not afraid to offer their own stories and to jump on board with me. My people. My village.

Above all of them, though, is the person who has literally held me up when I couldn't stand. The person who picked up all the pieces when I lay shattered on the ground. The person who saw me at my weakest and loved me more for it. The person that reminds me every day that I am all he needs. And that is my Jack. In a life where I couldn't imagine that this was happening to me, it was easy to forget that it was happening to him, too. As I complicated my grief with all the colorless varieties of self-pity, seeing me cry was his only weakness. This experience does not just happen to the women. It hits the men too, maybe in different ways, but they still feel the blow. Powerless in a world that they should be protecting. He somehow found the way to be there for me in a way that no one else could. Maybe that's what husbands do, or maybe I just have the best one on the entire planet.

These people said I was strong, and they were proud of me. But if everyone says that and you are crumbling on the inside, are you still strong? Or have you just fooled everyone? Is trying to put on a bold face acting strong? I don't know. I didn't know how to feel. I flip-flopped from being strong and knowing I could do this to being absolutely petrified. I didn't know what was going to happen. I didn't know how I was supposed to feel. Was I going to be proud of myself a year later? Two years later? Were *they* going to be proud of me? Either way, and for whatever it's worth, thank you.

CHAPTER 35

THE MERCK TOUR

Tomorrow is the day when I have to wake up, put on my clothes, and drive to RMA. It will be a normal day for everyone else driving around, but not for me. Tomorrow I will sit in that chair for possibly the last time, and they will draw my blood. The blood that will tell us if the procedure worked. If I was pregnant or if I wasn't. I had a gut feeling this morning that it wasn't going to work for some reason. I don't know why I felt that way. I just did. My negative thoughts started to creep back...my old friends. I thought I was so far from those feelings, but bad spells like this made me realize that they were always lurking, waiting for me to feel vulnerable. I'm not sure if it's my guarded brain playing tricks on me, after two years of disappointment, training me to think this way. I just feel sad. I try to think positively and look at the bright side. But my mind won't go there completely. I have to protect myself, prepare myself for the possibility that the implantation might not have worked.

Everyone around me felt excited for me. But "excited" didn't feel like the right word. The prospect was not exciting for me. There was too much on the line. IVF transfers at my age had a success rate of 60 percent, pretty good but by no means a given. My throat felt heavy, stress weighing me down. I didn't really know what to think. If this worked, then I was pregnant. If this worked, I had the chance to have two of my own children someday. I could start to feel happy again.

If it didn't, though, I had only one more chance left. I would have to confront all those people who believed I would succeed this time. I had to see the disappointment in Jack's eyes again. I had to hear everyone's pep talks and speeches again. I was too close to that time when I was lost to myself, and I didn't want to feel that way again. Maybe it's a classic progesterone bomb. *Who knows?* I was just tired and sad. I wanted more than this for myself. I wanted more than this for Jack. I wanted more than this for my mother, who had to watch grandchild after grandchild visit all her friends. I just wanted more.

Then I thought of Janine and everything she had told me. I kept remembering that picture she showed me. It gave me hope, knowing I had more than one option.

Still, on that day prior to the blood test, I just needed the hours to pass. With good news, I could start feeling whole again. I needed to stay positive.

I left work early since I couldn't concentrate on anything else. I started to feel some cramping in my lower stomach. I couldn't tell if it was my period or just my mind playing tricks on me. All I could think about was how devastating that would be; after coming all this way only to be no further than we were a year ago. I needed to do something to pass the time. So what did I do? I made soup. Don't ask me why. I guess I was just out of ideas. I thought chopping all the vegetables would distract me. So that's what I did. I started to make the worst soup that anyone's ever made.

As I walked toward the stove to stir my concoction, I felt something dripping between my legs. Chills went up my spine. I slowly slid my hand down the waistband of my leggings and felt for the bottom of my underwear. When I looked at my hand, there was blood on the tip of my finger. I couldn't breathe. I ran into the bathroom to take a closer look. Brownish blood seeped all over the toilet paper.

This was not happening. I ran to my phone to call the doctor. It was 3:53 p.m., and I knew they would be at work for only another seven minutes. A nurse picked up. I told her what had happened. She paused and asked me a few questions. She said not to panic. She said that this could happen. *Could happen?* What does that mean? Could happen if what? I didn't buy her cop-out response. She said to just wait until the blood test tomorrow. Again, I found myself alone with my thoughts, staring my greatest fear in the face.

After a restless night of sleep, it was barely 4:45 a.m. when I opened my eyes. I got up and jumped in the shower. This would be the most important day yet. The furthest we had gotten. The day we had been waiting for. I had to get to RMA by six. Getting the results would take a few hours, and I figured the earlier I got there, the earlier I would hear. The kicker was that today, Merck Pharmaceuticals, one of our biggest clients, was coming in for a huge tour of our facility and a lunch afterward. Of all days, this was the day they chose. I had no idea how I was going to keep my mind focused on the meeting when all I would be able to think about was getting that call. I had no choice, though.

The sky was tinted red as I drove toward RMA. I thought back to all those early mornings I had driven there and back for random testing. I pulled into the parking lot, took a deep breath, and walked in. Everything felt different. The hallways, the chairs, even the looks of the people that I passed. It was as if they all knew I was there today for a good reason. A really good reason. Putting the thought of my bloody underwear aside, I walked closer toward the truth.

They called my name as they had hundreds of times before. I walked in and sat in the chair as the nurse wrapped that rubber band around my arm to take my blood. She put the needle in and drew a vial's worth. For the first time, I couldn't bear to watch. She placed it on the table as she cleaned me up.

As she was talking a mile a minute to another nurse, I saw the vial start to roll toward the edge of the table. Before I could find my words, I watched it roll over the edge. She cursed as it hit the ground. "I'm sorry, darling, we are going to have to do it again."

My body was shaking, and I couldn't believe what was happening. Didn't she realize what this test meant? Just get this blood into the lab already! She repeated the blood test again, careful this time to secure it. And then off it went. The blood was officially off to testing. All I could do now was wait.

When I got to my office, all I could think about was when RMA was going to call. I started to analyze all the different times they had called me for results in the past. The timing. The tone of their voices. Trying to come up with a logical conclusion on when I would hear from them. I finally decided they would call somewhere between twelve and three. The Merck tour was starting at 10:30 a.m., followed by a lunch. What if I found out before? What if it was bad news? Should I take the call at that point or concentrate on the meeting and let the results go to voicemail? I worked through every scenario in my head. Yet I knew full well that I wouldn't have the slightest degree of self-control when RMA did call.

At 9:55 a.m., my phone rang, and the caller ID read RMA. I just sat there, stiff—like those dreams where you are trying to move your body but can't. I finally picked up the phone and swiped right to answer it. I could barely get out a timid hello as I gulped hard into the back of my throat. After a pause, I heard Nurse Adrienne's voice. My girl. "Your results are in and so, yeah...you're pregnant."

The phone slid from my hands and onto the floor. I started to laugh. I laughed so hard that I couldn't speak. Not the reaction I pictured myself having, but that's what happened. I stumbled to pick up the phone from the floor to talk to her again. It felt like all the blood in my body had rushed to my head, and I felt drunk with emotion. I kept thanking her profusely.

She said that I had to come back in the next day for another blood test. They wanted to make sure the HCG (Human Chorionic Gonadotropin) levels doubled in order to confirm that I had a viable pregnancy. Then we would come back in a few weeks to hear the heartbeat.

But none of that mattered today. What mattered was that I'd heard the words that I had been wanting to hear for two years: "You...are...pregnant."

I sat there for a few minutes alone with myself, basking in the news. It was time to tell Jack. My fingers shook as I dialed his number. When he answered, he could barely say hello, knowing exactly why I was calling. Before he could say another word, I interrupted:

"It worked! Jack, it worked. I'm pregnant. We're having a baby."

Only silence filled the other end, but it spoke a thousand words. I knew he was crying. I wanted to crawl through the phone lines and hold his face in my hands.

I heard his voice quiver: "I love you. I love you so much. We're going to have a family."

I hung up the phone and ran into Vince's office. He stood up immediately, knowing I had heard something by the way I stormed in. "It worked!"

He dropped back down in his chair. He put his face in his hands and started to cry. He cried harder than I had ever seen a man cry before. Gasping for breaths. A reaction that I never saw coming. A year's worth of weight lifted off his shoulders. The shock of relief wracking his body. A raw display of emotion. I realized how much hurt and sadness he had been carrying for all of us. His own happiness suppressed by his concern for me. He was finally able to let his guard down. I walked up and hugged him from behind as he cried. My Vince. My twin.

I then proceeded to tell just a few people: my older brother, his wife, Grace, my parents, Jack's parents, Jaci, Dani, Sarah in Colorado, Marla in London, and a client who happened to call in the middle of all of it. Okay, so maybe I couldn't stop telling people. But you know what, when you've had enough bad days, you're allowed to celebrate the good ones. We had done it. We could all finally breathe again. And now it was time—for the Merck tour.

When I got home that night, I went to my bathroom cabinet. I had been saving one last pregnancy test. I told myself I would wait until I knew it would read positive. I was determined to never read a negative on one of those things again. I took it out of the wrapper and peed on it. Even though I knew what it would say, I still had that feeling of dread in the pit of my stomach. Within seven seconds, the word "Pregnant" came up.

It came up so fast and so clear that it made me laugh at how many times I thought I was pregnant with imaginary lines and delayed results. I left the test on the counter so that Jack would see it when he walked in. It may have been two years late, and it may not have had the surprise factor that most reveals have, but it read positive, and it was ours. And that's all that mattered. We were having a baby.

CHAPTER 36

MY HEARTBEAT SONG

I'm happy. So happy. Really, I am. I think. This is what we wanted. But the thing is I go back and forth between being relieved and realizing how fast it could be taken away from me. Is that normal? I try to stay reserved, so reserved that sometimes it feels like I'm convincing myself to be excited. I guess it just feels like it all happened so fast. Three weeks ago, I was crying in my car wondering if this would ever happen for me, and here I am, pregnant, waiting for a heartbeat check, with everyone around me expecting me to do a happy dance. Maybe it doesn't feel real yet.

I've dreamt about writing this chapter from the moment I started. I hoped that I would get to a point where I would be able to write about how this process finally worked and how magical it would be. But I don't quite feel like that. I haven't cried yet either. Is that weird? I never had that ah-ha moment. The one where my mom and I are screaming and hugging. I can't say I'm nervous. I'm not. I feel good about where everything is. I'm just not bursting at the seams, and I feel bad about that. I have been trying to pretend so people don't think I'm ungrateful. Trust me: I understand what an incredible blessing this is. It's just that my life has been on pause for two years, and now suddenly, someone pushed the fast-forward button and here I am. Happy. So happy. Really, I am. I think.

I had never gone to RMA for a "good reason." Pulling up today, pregnant, had an entirely different feel. I was anxious to hear the heartbeat, hoping it would give me the closure I needed. A part of me felt guilty I had made it through while so many were left behind. Jack immediately went to check us in, while I just waited quietly. Taking it all in. Seeing what I had seen one hundred times but through different eyes.

When I went in for my blood test, the room was crowded with people waiting. The girl next to me was looking down at her arms searching for an unbruised vein for her next blood test. The girl next to her sat staring into space. But it was the girl in front of me who caught my eye. She wore a Giants football sweatshirt and leggings. Her hair was pulled up in a tight bun. Nothing out of the ordinary. Her face, though, I will never forget. When the nurse came over to her, she said, "Yeah, I'm back." Despair was written all over her face. So many emotions filled my body. It was like I was looking at an old photo album. What I'd won didn't feel fair. She would do anything to be in my shoes, and I was sitting here, selfishly unsure about how I was feeling.

As we waited to go into the ultrasound room, I couldn't stop noticing the faces of the women around me, women I had avoided eye contact with for months, not wanting them to know we were failing. Now I fixated on their faces, desperate for them not to know that we had succeeded. When the nurse called our name, I stood up and took a deep breath. It was time.

The doctor was late coming into the room, leaving Jack and I in a silent limbo. We would share a quick nervous smile and then go back to our own thoughts. I wondered what his were. Was he imagining me pregnant? Maybe daydreaming of his new life? I just stared at my underwear lying calmly in my shoe, as I had so many times before. But this time was different.

The doctor came in and got right down to business. She knew we were anxious to see. She lubed up the wand and slowly inserted it. She moved it around, searching for the little embryo. As she looked, she kept saying that it was early, and the embryo might be hard to see at this point. It sounded like an excuse to me. But then she paused and stopped moving the wand. Her eyes widened. "See that little moving dot? That's it! That's the heartbeat."

I grabbed Jack's hand tighter than ever before. We were staring at our baby, little heart beating away. It was surreal—a little life starting in there. The doctor printed out some pictures and left the room. Jack and I kept hugging and laughing in disbelief. I felt the light at the end of the tunnel pulling me through. Could we really be having a baby?

When we walked out, I had to make a quick stop in the bathroom. Jack took off because he had to catch a train back into the city. When I pulled up my skirt, I felt a weird sensation on my upper thighs. I pulled down my underwear and found blood everywhere. It was spreading all over my clothes, and it kept coming out. My heart stopped, and I started to panic. I grabbed the wall of the stall as I sat on the toilet. I started to breathe harder and harder as I kept wiping myself down, hoping for the blood to stop.

I wrapped myself in my coat and ran back into the office and told them what happened. They said they would have the doctor come back out. As I sat there alone, I had a horrible feeling. I knew it had felt too good to be true. I was silly for thinking that would be it for me. I couldn't move. I felt stiff. I was too upset to cry, even as every bad scenario raced through my head.

Nurse Adrienne came running out. She looked me deep in the eyes and said to stay calm. She personally walked me back in as if to push anyone out of the way that even remotely tried to delay me. She took me to a more private room that contained another ultrasound machine. She waited with me until the doctor came in.

Having her there meant everything to me. When the doctor walked in, he came right over to the table and put the wand in and started to look around. That little fighter's heart was still beating away. I let out a sigh of relief. The doctor explained that a pocket of blood could've been aggravated by the ultrasound and released. The shock of seeing that blood was the most frightened I had been through this entire process, a harsh reminder that I was only ever one mishap away from being back to where I started. He said the hormone levels were substantially increasing and the baby's heartbeat was strong. But there was something that I couldn't let go of, and I couldn't quite put my finger on it.

From then on, I felt numb. I didn't know how to feel. Something was holding me back from full-blown happiness, and I didn't know how to make it better. Everyone around me was excited.

They wanted to go shopping for baby clothes, and they wanted to scream and jump up and down. But I wasn't feeling that way. I almost felt like I was still mourning what we had gone through. Maybe I was in shock that it worked. Maybe I was left feeling like the other shoe was about to drop. Maybe I felt more connected to the person I was before this. I couldn't just turn a switch and forget all those heavy emotions I felt. It was like that feeling you get when you are fighting with your husband, and he apologizes and you know you have to snap out of it, but you still feel angry.

I was also really nauseous. Everyone around me seemed happy about that. It showed that there was a healthy baby in there! Other mothers kept saying how they loved it and how they thought it was their baby giving them signs. I didn't feel signs. I just felt nauseous—nauseous and tired. And emotionless. Was this normal? I didn't know who to ask because I was embarrassed that I felt this way. Maybe I was just not that kind of mother. Was this postpartum? Prepartum? Was I not going to love my own child?

One Tuesday afternoon, when work was slow, I decided to go home early. Jack was going to be working really late, and I thought it would be a good chance to do some chores I'd put off. When I got home, I started to clear up the random piles that had been gathering in various corners of the house, bills that needed to be paid, and mail that I had to sort through. Then I started doing the dishes and putting them away in the cabinets. Then I started to rearrange the cabinets. And then I became a complete and utter psychopath: cleaning out the closets and switching my winter clothes over to my spring clothes. You know because it's February. I dusted the tops of the lights that had been gathering dust for months, annoying the shit out of me every time I looked at them. This neurotic pace went on and on for hours. It felt slightly insane. I kept avoiding our dining room. I'd glance in and then steer myself in another direction, rushing past it as I completed my rounds of frantic cleaning and organizing.

Before I realized it, it was eight o'clock. I couldn't believe it. I walked toward the dining room and plopped myself down on one of the chairs. I let out a huge sigh as I fell exhausted onto the cushion. As I sat there, I couldn't peel my eyes away from the cabinet in the corner. I knew what was inside. Without thinking, I counted to three and got up. I opened the cabinet hastily and took out what was inside. I opened the top of a huge plastic bag and poured out its contents: a year's worth of needles I never used, medications I had been saving, random types of gauzes and ointments that had been separated from their original boxes long ago. As I rummaged through the assorted supplies, the emotions came flooding back. I started to breathe heavily. I felt my heart starting to race, and I had to put my two hands on the edge of the table for balance. I brought my head down to my arms as I fell to my knees. And then I did something that I never saw coming. I started to sob. I cried so savagely that if anyone heard me, they would have thought someone had died. I curled up on the ground, my face pressed tight to the rug. I cried harder than I ever remember crying before. I don't even know why. Seeing all those needles again, the realization of what it had all meant sprawled out on the table. Maybe I opened the door again. Or maybe, just maybe I was closing it.

I let myself lie there for a bit, an intimate moment that I hadn't yet had with myself. When I knew I was ready, I pulled myself up off the floor, dusted myself off, and gathered all the needles up again. I put them in a large plastic container and wrapped it with duct tape. I walked out to the garage. I held the bag in my arms one last time and then threw it away. I closed the top of the bin and slowly backed away. As I walked into the house, I wanted to look back, but I didn't.

Instead, I closed the door behind me and smiled. It was time to forgive myself for moving on, to release myself from a life that no longer defined me. Relinquishing the worry that held me back, I took a deep breath and looked down at my stomach as I rolled my hand across it. It was no longer about me. It was about him.

CHAPTER 37

TO MY IVF GIRLS

My dear IVF girls. This chapter's for you.

I know the journey can be hard. I know the journey can be unfair. And I know the journey can be flat-out unbearable. But hold on. Hold on harder than you ever have before. If you're deep in it, if you're sitting at home looking at Facebook, feeling like the only woman on earth without kids. If you just got another disappointing result from the doctor. If it feels like you will never feel like yourself again. You are not alone.

No matter what your details are or how messy the process has gotten, I know you can do this. The fact that you picked up this book and read it means that you're longing for answers. You're fighting the good fight. I promise you at the end of all of this, you'll learn things about yourself that you never knew were inside you. Never give up hope. Never.

This book shares my personal story, but there are thousands of others out there—most far worse than mine, I'm sure. I know the details are different, but we share the one thing that draws us all together. Bravery. Bravery that comes from looking your biggest fear in the face and diving in anyway. Bravery in refusing to let disappointment be the last feeling you feel. Bravery to show up to the baby showers, the parties, or even just work every day with a smile on your face. But most of all, the courage to fight a battle that no one has taught you how to fight.

I don't know how your journey will end. But I do know this. You will be a mother someday if you want to be, no matter what package it comes in. One thing I've learned is that being a mother means so much more than just getting pregnant. And everything you're going through now will make you the best fucking mother on the planet. One day, you'll look your baby in the eyes, and it will feel like the only baby you were ever meant to have, and you won't care if it came from you, a donor, an orphanage, or a goddamn coconut tree.

You're not alone. I'm here for you. Sarah is here for you. Martine is here for you. Janine is here for you. So are Heather, Francine, Ashley, and Tara. There are thousands of others, too. Women who you'll never know, silently rooting for you every time they think of their own story. So, for right now, take a deep breath and feel their strength. Look doubt in the face when it's trying to push you into the hole and yell at the top of your lungs: not today! You've got this, and I'm so proud of you. Just wait and see. This world has funny ways of making your dreams come true.

For the rest of you—freeze your eggs, for God's sake.

↗ CHAPTER 38 ↖

OBGYN-*LMNOP*

The sun shone brightly on this March day as I drove up to the OBGYN, one year from the start of my IVF journey. As I pulled into the parking lot, everything felt familiar, like I had been there a thousand times. This was my turn. I had made it. I had crossed to the island where the normal women get to go, where they were all waiting to cheer my arrival. I was a survivor. A heroine even.

When I heard my name called, I walked into the room and sat down. There were no gowns to be worn or wands attached to computer screens. No awards on the walls or tissues on the counter. Just a chair and a laptop. When the doctor came in, she ran through some questions as she looked through my form. I wondered if she would ask me about our journey. She asked if I had ever been pregnant before. She asked about how I was feeling. She even asked what seemed to be the most important question of all: was I allergic to latex? But nothing about the IVF. I guess it didn't matter anymore. I was just, simply, caught up. My finish line, everyone else's starting gate. I found myself wanting to scream out loud, "So nobody wants to hear my story? NOBODY?" I'm not sure what I expected or why. I didn't want a medal or anything. Maybe I just wanted someone to understand. Feel a part of something. I was proud. As I walked back out to the parking lot, suddenly everything felt unfamiliar. I didn't feel like I was part of something as special as I thought. But the truth was, I was a part of something special. Just not there.

I got in my car and started to drive, past the signs for the Holland Tunnel, past the exit to my house. I pulled into the parking lot like I had so many times and turned off the car. I was at a place that would never forget: RMA. I sat there for what seemed like hours. I watched as the women filed in and out of the doors, limping out in their pajama pants, with their red faces hidden under their winter coats. There was more behind those bloodshot eyes. They may have felt battered today, but they were bold. They were brave.

I looked past my stomach, which had just started to show, and down to the steering wheel into the empty space toward my feet. As I fixated on them, my mind played back every emotion from the year before. A warmth came over me. I felt blessed. Not just for the outcome, but for having gone through this experience. For everything it taught me about myself. For exposing me to a level of human awareness that will forever change the way I treat people. And for showing me the amazing strength and kindness that is within us and around us if you are lucky enough for the opportunity to open your eyes to see it.

In the darkness, I noticed the outline of my shoes, fresh out of battle, with soles that rushed in and out of the same doors as these women today. The toes were stained white from the snow of the winter before. The tops were stretched out from the tugging of pulling them off and on. They represented a struggle that only we can truly understand. It hit me, right then and there, we are not alone. None of us. Everything that we have been through will bond us forever. And we *will* be better for it. Those women who come after us will be able to benefit from our stories the way we did from the women who came before us.

I wanted to look up and say to each woman coming out of those doors that it would be okay. I wanted to tell them they were not alone and that they would never be again. But they wouldn't understand. Not yet. They were too enveloped in their own reality. But they'll get there. As we all did. All I could do for now was sit there and look down at my shoes, like I had so many times before. They may have looked worn. And they certainly wouldn't pass Tribeca standards. But they walked a path that only a few of us have walked—a journey that no one can take away from me. They were mine. Bold. Brave...and underwear free.

EPILOGUE

October 6, 2018. The waiting room was packed with grandparents, aunts, uncles, and cousins anxiously awaiting your arrival. It was 7:39 p.m. when I caught the first glimpse of your little face. "It's a boy." I heard Daddy proudly shout. You were eight pounds one ounce with a head full of bushy brown hair that everyone in the hospital was talking about. As they placed you in my arms, you stopped crying. A person I had never met but had always known. I realized, as you stared back into my eyes, that I hadn't been the only one fighting. A moment you will never remember. A moment I will never forget. You are, and will always be, worth it all.

THINGS I'VE LEARNED ALONG THE WAY

Don't blame people for saying the wrong things.

Don't come to your own conclusions.

Take one day at a time.

I have no idea the correct usage of commas.

Get the Fallopian tube test!! I've learned that some practices don't do this as a standard procedure. DO IT! It can save you a lot of heartache *and money* if it works.

Talk about it with your family and friends. You have nothing to be ashamed of.

It only takes one.

It's not your fault.

Don't miss the cup.

You are not a human incubator. You are someone's mother. There's no gray area.

Throw away your home pregnancy tests. *I mean it, you!*

Blame everything on your hormones. You've earned it.

GET THE GENETIC TESTING!

Don't write your ending before it happens.

Don't be afraid to change your ending.

Don't ever give up hope. EVER.

ACKNOWLEDGMENTS

To everyone who had their lives sprawled out on my pages: thank you for helping me paint the real-life picture of this experience to support the bigger cause.

For all the women who opened up to me about their IVF stories: you helped me to see clearer the emotions behind endings that were different than mine. I drew strength from your courage. You will always be in my heart and in my soul.

John Paine: for believing in me and this project and for your professional edit. You pushed me to be better, and the book came to life because of it.

To all my family and friends not specifically mentioned but that were there to support me through IVF as well as writing this book, thank you. After a solid laugh when you realized I actually knew how to read, your support and excitement was contagious, and

I appreciate your loyalty in helping to do all you could to make my dreams come true.

Scott Alpaugh: for having my back whenever I needed it. Whether it was connecting me with some extraordinary people, or just being there for me to vent, your energy and devotion to me and this project will never be forgotten. I wish I could write your entire acknowledgment in mini letters, but I'm not allowed.

Scribe Media: for your support and expertise along the way. I simply could not have done it without you. Your passionate team inspired me every day. Emily Anderson, thank you for keeping the boat afloat and for answering my crazy emails no matter how many I sent. Erin Tyler, your cover design was brilliant, and I loved every moment I got to talk with you about it. Who knew a shoe could have so many colors and angles! Manolo sisters forever! A special thanks to Jenny Shipley, you were not only my editor but also my therapist at times. Thank you for giving me the confidence to keep fighting for what I believed in. Your expertise was inspiring, and I felt honored to work on this project with you.

Anthony Ramondo: for your patience, willingness, and friendship throughout this process. The respect and trust I have for you are immense, and I felt so honored to have had the opportunity to have your guidance in these unchartered territories of book publishing.

My beta readers, Debra Costanza, Katherine Schellenger, Stefanie Werring, Sarah Treadway, Alex Cassou, and Joseph Russo: You were the first to read this manuscript at its earliest draft. Unleashing it into the wild scared me to death, but your feedback inspired and challenged me to be better. Thank you for taking the time out of your busy lives to help me. It meant more to me than you could ever know.

Marla Russo: You are always there for me no matter the task. You show your love for me every day. For that I can never thank you enough. You're my sister, my confidante, and my friend. Thanks for your PR advice along the way. It meant a lot in those confusing moments.

Jaclyn Costanza: for your constant support throughout this journey. You spent many a late night with me, reading random chapters and giving me feedback as we laughed over red wine. Thank you for being my cheerleader and for believing in me always. Verbals, baby!

Sarah Treadway: for always being there for me. Your support and guidance through this journey are something I will never be able to explain. I quite simply could not have gotten through it without you. The place you have sealed in my heart will always be with me.

Eve Russo: for bravely letting me tell my story at the expense of your own. Your selflessness and support through this process is unmatched and truly appreciated. It takes a strong confident woman to do that. From the bottom of my heart, thank you.

Nolan Russo: for always believing in me no matter how consumed in it I became. There was never a time I could talk about it too much. Your love for me is selfless, pure, and unconditional. I carry it with me always.

Dr. Scott: I am completely and utterly indebted to you and your practice. Besides being completely star struck every time you walked into the room, your compassion, understanding, and deep passion for your patients shined through in every conversation you had with us. I will never be able to describe the gratitude I have in my heart for all you do for this field. You will always be a part of our family.

Nurse Adrienne: you made me feel less alone. Hearing your voice was soothing to me every single time, even on the bad days. You had my back from the start, and your kindness and willingness to let us into your heart meant so much to my family as we embarked on this impossible journey.

Danielle Alpaugh: for editing with me in between being a lawyer, a wife, and a mother of two. The time you gave me will never be forgotten as will your friendship. Thank you for translating my writing to English. *"I know what you're trying to say, but that's not really a word."* Bottom line: YOU FREAKIN' SMART! Thank you for helping me through this process and through my journey.

Linda Russo, my mother: for your constant support pushing me forward. Thank you for the confidence you gave me, the late-night calls, the soft pushes to keep going and everything in between. You picked up the phone no matter the hour when I had a chapter to read you or needed an opinion. Your honesty made me step outside my comfort zone and never settle. Your love for me is fierce. You taught me more about being a mother this year than ever before.

My husband: for giving me my "Walt Whitman" time and for supporting me in this dream. Thank you for your willingness to share your story at the expense of your own privacy. You talked me through many overwhelming writer's blocks and editing challenges. This was new territory for both of us but exciting all the same. Your love for me is boundless, and I appreciate you jumping onboard with me on this.

My son: for giving up some of your mommy time to get this ever-so-important message out. Seeing your sleeping face in the rocker next to me inspired me to keep writing to help other women live out their motherhood dreams as you have helped me live out mine. You will always be at the heart of everything I do.

ABOUT THE AUTHOR

BRETT RUSSO was born and raised in New Jersey. She graduated with a degree in business management from Bucknell University, where she also met her future husband.

After graduation, Brett found her passion working beside her twin brother and father for her family's printing company of which she is now the chief executive officer. She married her husband in 2015, and together they fought the hardest battle of their lives with their journey through IVF.

Brett lives in New Jersey with her husband and their one-year-old son, who enjoys meatloaf and responding with "Nah" every time his mom asks for a kiss.

Made in the USA
Middletown, DE
10 November 2020

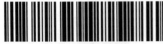